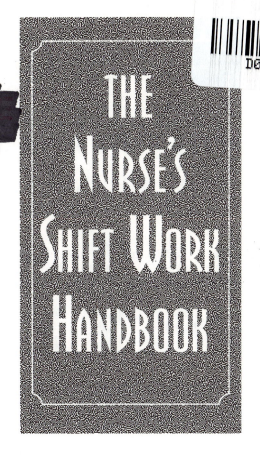

THE NURSE'S SHIFT WORK HANDBOOK

RUTH R. ALWARD, Ed.D., R.N.

AND

TIMOTHY H. MONK, Ph.D.

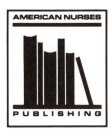

AMERICAN NURSES
PUBLISHING

American Nurses Publishing is the publishing program
of the American Nurses Foundation, an affiliate organization
of the American Nurses Association.

Ruth R. Alward, Ed.D., R.N., is president of Nurse Executive Associates, Inc. of Washington, D.C., which provides consultation, education, and research services to the nursing profession. Dr. Alward became interested in studying nurses' adaptations to shift work when she was first exposed to the theory of circadian rhythms in the 1970s. Some of her fascination with the subject was driven by memories of the difficulty she had adapting to shift work early in her nursing career. Her shift work research studies during the past 10 years have included several in collaboration with Dr. Monk.

Dr. Alward co-authored *The Nurse's Guide to Marketing* (1991), and has published articles in national and international nursing journals. She is editor of Delmar Publisher's "Professional Reference Series for Nurse Administrators and Managers," and has served on the editorial advisory board for the *Journal of Nursing Administration* since 1983.

Timothy H. Monk, Ph.D., is associate professor of psychiatry at the University of Pittsburgh School of Medicine, and director of the university's Human Chronobiology Research Program. Dr. Monk first became interested in nursing shift work issues when he collaborated in a large-scale study of night shift nurses at Northwick Park Hospital in London in the mid-1970s.

Since then, Dr. Monk has written numerous articles and chapters on shift work topics, and has been involved in three other shift work books: *Hours of Work: Temporal Factors in Work Scheduling* (co-edited with Dr. Simon Folkard in 1985), *How to Make Shift Work Safe and Productive* (written in 1988), and *Making Shiftwork Tolerable* (co-authored with Dr. Folkard in 1992). Additionally, Dr. Monk has served on the International Commission on Occupational Health's Scientific Committee on Shiftwork since 1983, and was recently appointed editor of the *Shiftwork International Newsletter*.

ISBN 1-55810-087-3

Published by American Nurses Publishing
600 Maryland Avenue, S.W.
Suite 100 West
Washington, D.C. 20024

NP-82   4M   11/93

To Sam and Fran, for their loving support,
and to the millions of nurses who
burn the midnight oil.

Contents

Introduction

History of Shift Work

S hift work has existed for centuries. According to Scherrer's (1981) historical review, traffic congestion in ancient Rome was reduced by restricting deliveries in the city to the night hours, which put most of the delivery service sector on the "graveyard" shift. In order to ensure fresh products for morning shoppers, bakers have toiled through the last half of the night for hundreds of years. Seven-hundred-year-old European guild records contain complaints that night work reduced workers' efficiency (Mott et al., 1965). Because of workers' protests and lighting difficulties, the industrial sector made minimal use of night workers before the Industrial Revolution and the invention of electric light. In the service sector, however, evening and night work have always been required of those who guard the safety and well-being of others, such as nurses, soldiers, sailors, police officers, fire fighters, and security guards.

Although industrial night work for women was forbidden by the International Labor Organization (ILO — a United Nations agency) [U.S. Congress, 1991], exceptions have generally been made for night shift nurses and many other female workers, making the "ban" more of a goal than a reality. The United States has not ratified the ILO conventions prohibiting night work for women. During the 1970s, the U.S. Equal Employment Opportunity Commission found laws against night work by women discriminatory under Title VII of the Civil Rights Act, and all U.S. states that previously had laws forbidding women to work at night repealed them.

Increased accident rates and decreased productivity often are associated with night work. As a result of the Three Mile Island nuclear power station incident (which involved the near meltdown of a nuclear reactor, primarily because of workers' errors at night) [Mitler et al., 1988], shift work problems have been given more attention by the mass media. Since Three Mile Island, major U.S. newspapers and weekly news magazines have regularly featured stories on the dangers of a chronically fatigued work force in the health care, nuclear power, and transportation industries. In an introduction to the proceedings of an international symposium on shift work, Reinberg, Vieux, and Andlauer (1981) label as "dangerous illusions" the widely held assumptions that all people can work voluntarily at any time of the 24-hour day and can tolerate shift work equally well.

Nurse Shift Workers

Shift work is an integral part of nursing. Most nurses are either shift workers now or have been shift workers in the past. By *shift work* we mean a work schedule in which regular work hours fall outside of the typical 7:00 a.m. to 6:00 p.m. time frame, and which includes evening and night work assigned on a fixed or rotating basis. In the United States, approximately three-fourths of the estimated 1.6 million employed registered nurses work in hospitals or nursing homes (Moses, 1990), all of which require staffing 24-hours-per-day, seven-days-per-week.

There are many different problems associated with shift work, including sleep and sleepiness, anxiety and interpersonal conflicts, and loss of good mental and physical health. Sleep and sleepiness problems result from disruptions of the nurse's biological clock, which can interfere both with off-shift sleep and on-shift performance. Anxiety and interpersonal difficulties arise from the shift worker's schedule, which conflicts with the day-oriented, nine-to-five, five-days-a-week work pattern of the rest of society (and often, more importantly, of the nurse's own spouse and children). Additionally, these conflicts can lead to feelings of loneliness, alienation, and professional isolation. At both the emotional and biological levels, the stress of coping with shift work can lead to ill health, particularly in the areas of sleep disorders, gastrointestinal distress, depressive symptoms, and substance abuse.

Nurses' Shift Work Adaptation Program

Although there is a growing body of literature on shift work, very little has been published in the nursing arena that provides coping strategies appropriate to the health care environment. This book is written specifically for nurses and nurse managers, though we hope that other health care workers involved in around-the-clock shifts also will find it useful.

The primary aim of this book is to help nurse shift workers understand the physiological, psychological, and sociological factors that contribute to their shift work problems, and to encourage them to undertake adaptation programs that help them to more effectively cope with shift work. In turn, nurses can then teach coping strategies to clients, patients, and family members who are shift workers. There is no quick fix for shift work problems, but there are scientific facts that lay the foundation for an educational program appropriate for the nurse shift worker, which we call the Nurses' Shift Work Adaptation Program (NSWAP). The goal of the NSWAP is to assist nurses in implementing personal and professional coping strategies that are appropriate to their own shift work situations.

A secondary aim of this book is to educate nurses who are responsible for staff development, recruitment and retention of nursing staff, and development of work schedules and staffing plans so that they can use the NSWAP information to facilitate shift work assignments for staff members.

Additionally, through the information presented in this book, we hope to educate and motivate nurse researchers. There is a strong need for academic nursing departments and clinical nurse researchers to address shift work issues and conduct studies of coping strategies and shift systems that might help optimize nurses' performance and well-being.

Structure of the Book

There are 10 chapters in this book. After the general introduction to shift work in the nursing profession presented in Chapter 1, subsequent chapters provide the background nurses will need to understand the etiology of the shift work problem. Chapter 2 focuses on biological factors, introducing the biological clock that governs the daily cycles of rest and activity, and which plays a significant role in complicating the life of the shift worker. Results of relevant laboratory and field studies are summarized. Chapter 3 deals with social, professional, and domestic issues related to shift work. Chapter 4 focuses on the health of the nurse shift worker, discussing problem areas such as the gastrointestinal tract, the menstrual cycle, pregnancy, and psychological status. Chapter 5 addresses the sleep of shift workers, discussing how sleep is measured and quantified into different stages and depths, napping, and changes in sleep patterns related to age. Chapter 6 deals with performance at night, discussing circadian performance in general and night nurse performance in particular. Chapter 7 focuses on the assessment and planning phases of the NSWAP development. Goal setting, time management, and the assessment of individual shift work strengths and weaknesses are included. Chapter 8 specifies actions that nurses can take to help them cope with shift work problems. This is the essence of the NSWAP. Chapter 9 discusses the nurse administrator's role in selecting, scheduling, educating, and supporting shift nurses. This discussion includes recommendations for making shift work systems less disruptive and the nursing staff more productive and safe — for both themselves and their patients. Chapter 10 reviews shift work as it relates to national and international health care policies, nursing association policies, and current management policies. An Epilogue, a Glossary of common shift work terms, and a list of References conclude the book.

— Chapter 1 —

Shift Work and Nursing

Introduction

Shift work is not a new concept, particularly in the health care professions. What has changed over the years is the number of people unavoidably affected by nonstandard work schedules. In the past, individuals who did not work during the day were often a highly self-selected group — actively wanting and expecting to do shift work. If the unusual hours did not suit them, they simply switched to occupations that permitted day work. In recent times, however, so many services and industrial processes have sprung up that require around-the-clock coverage, and so many good day jobs have disappeared, that the "exit option" is less available to the shift worker. When a worker is committed to a shift work position (whether for financial, domestic, or professional reasons), it is often difficult to find a comparable day work alternative. Consequently, the millions of people affected by shift work are now trying even harder to find ways to survive the difficulties of shift work.

Estimates vary as to the exact number of people employed in shift work positions, but approximately one-fifth of the work force in the United States works some form of shift schedule or system. In 1985, one-third of all dual-income couples with children had at least one spouse doing shift work (U.S. Congress, 1991). The percentage of nurses and health care workers engaged in shift work is undoubtedly considerably higher than the percentage of women shift workers in general. One government source (Mellor, 1986) estimates that

1

27% of 2,303,000 hospital workers (not including RNs) worked evening, night, or rotating shifts. In the health assessment and treating occupations category, which includes RNs, 31.3% were involved in some form of shift work.

Firm estimates of the current number of registered nurses involved in shift work are not available. The U.S. Public Health Service's Division of Nursing has not collected shift work data in its quadrennial National Sample Survey of Registered Nurses. In 1990, the Hospital Nursing Personnel Survey conducted by the American Hospital Association's Center for Nursing found that 31.2% of registered nurses worked a fixed day shift, 18.3% worked a fixed evening shift, and 18.0% worked a fixed night shift. Almost one-third of all hospital nurses (32.6%) worked a rotating shift (American Hospital Association, 1992). A 1985 survey of registered nurses employed in nursing homes reported that over 32% of RNs worked fixed evening or night shifts; another 9% worked rotating shifts (Jones et al., 1987).

Shift Systems

We commonly refer to the nurse's scheduled period of daily work as a *shift*. *Shift systems* are defined by several characteristics:

- the length of the work period per day (for example, an 8-hour shift, a 10-hour shift, or a 12-hour shift);
- the beginning and ending times of the shift (7:00 a.m. to 3:30 p.m., for example);
- the regularity or irregularity of the shift occurring at the same time in the 24-hour day (fixed vs. rotating shifts); and
- the speed at which rotational changes occur (rapid or slow rotation).

Rotation patterns are generally referred to as *rapid* if one or two periods are worked before changing to another shift, and as *comparatively rapid* if the limit is three or four shifts before a change. *Slow rotation* involves two or more consecutive weeks on one shift. A *weekly rotation* involves between five and seven consistent shifts before changing to a different work period. *Permanent* or *fixed shift* schedules seldom change. Many shift systems are so irregular that they defy categorization; one could argue that they are really nonsystems.

There are no known descriptive data on the number of nurses working in each of the various shift systems (and nonsystems) used in hospitals, nursing homes, and other health care organizations providing continuous nursing service. We do know that nurse managers use rotating shifts to supplement the ranks of permanent evening and night shift nurses. Additional compensation for shift work is almost universal in nursing organizations, with night workers generally receiving a greater differential payment than evening workers. Rotations are not commonly made to all three shifts in one week. Within one week, however, many nurses do rotate between days and evenings or between days and nights. In a very limited number of situations, no permanent shift workers are employed because of organizational policies (see Chapter 10). In many nursing organizations, when an adequate supply of fixed shift nurses can be hired, nurses only work rotating shifts to cover for unscheduled staff absences or emergencies.

In decentralized organizations, shift work policies are frequently determined on the nursing unit level. This process produces a great variety of shift systems within some large hospitals, where shift continua can range from self-scheduling and irregular assignment to very rigid cyclical patterns, and from rotating shift patterns to fixed shift patterns. Collective bargaining agreements may specify various aspects of a shift system. For example, rotational limits may be based on a nurse's seniority, and mandatory days off may be specified before and after night duty.

Nursing organizations also can exhibit great variety in scheduling hours of work and days off. Nurses commonly work a variety of duty periods, from 7½ to 13 hours per shift, in addition to a variety of short or part-time shifts. Although a 1990 survey found that slightly over two-thirds of hospital RNs (67.4%) worked eight-hour shifts, this percentage had dropped from 78.5% in 1988. During this same two-year period, the percentage of RNs working 12-hour shifts increased from 17.4% to 28.5%. The number of hospital RNs working 10-hour shifts dropped slightly from 2.7% to 2.5%. This survey found that 67.5% of hospital RNs worked fixed shifts of days, evenings, or nights, and that 32.6% worked some type of rotating shift (McMurtry, 1992).

As the number of nurses who work 12-hour shifts increases, there is a concurrent increase in the amount of rapid rotation and in sleep patterns resembling those of rapid rotation shift workers. A nurse who is working three or four 12-hour shifts in a week may work one or two consecutive nights and then have a night or two off before returning to the night shift. Even if this nurse works a fixed

3

night shift, the pattern resembles rapid rotation if the nurse reverts to night sleep on off-duty days. Rarely would the 12-hour shift nurse work five consecutive nights unless he or she was on a seven-on/seven-off shift system, or was holding a second nursing position that also involved night work.

To minimize desynchronized physiological rhythms, most European countries favor rotating schedules over fixed schedules, thereby spreading the night work burden over more of the work force. The number of consecutive night shifts assigned to each nurse may be restricted, resulting in the use of rapid rotation schedules that limit consecutive night shifts to three or less. In contrast, many North American nursing organizations favor weekly rotation or slow rotations of two weeks or more.

The rotational patterns most commonly used by nursing organizations in the U.S. are not described in any nursing literature the authors could find, although some studies have investigated the 8-hour and 12-hour shift length options. The literature reports great dissatisfaction with nursing work assignments and scheduling, including shift rotation practices; however, little nursing research has focused on optimal shift rotation patterns for nurses.

Shift Work Problems

Ask shift workers what their biggest problem is, and you will most likely receive the same answer — sleep. One example involves the case study of a recent patient at a sleep clinic. Jane is a 45-year-old registered nurse who worked permanent night shifts in an intensive care unit while she completed a master's program in nursing administration. New degree in hand, she accepted a critical care assistant director's position on the night shift. Jane's problem was acute sleepiness from about 3:00 a.m. to 5:00 a.m., when she sometimes resorted to taking a surreptitious nap on a sofa in the director's office. Since graduation, her work environment had changed from one with much stimulation and a need for all-night vigilance, to one with some monotony at the worst time for her biological rhythms. It was no coincidence that Jane's sleepiness problem surfaced as she entered her forties, and the fact that she had a new husband who wanted her to sleep at night on nonworking days only exacerbated her problem. As we will discuss in later chapters, both advancing age and domestic commitments can make it more difficult to cope successfully with shift work.

While Jane's problem involved sleep coming earlier than she wanted, Sarah's problem was that she could not sleep when she did want to. Sarah was a 24-year-old RN working 10 night rotations in charge of three psychiatric units. When she tried to sleep during the day, significant problems arose. Living in a house with three other nurse roommates led to much commotion on their various days off and, of course, the telephone rang, ambulances shrieked, and kids shouted in the neighbors' yards. Although Sarah was usually in bed by 8:30 a.m., it was impossible for her to sleep longer than five hours however long she stayed in bed. Then, of course, at 11:00 p.m. she desperately wanted to go to bed instead of to work. With coffee and an occasional Ritalin, Sarah managed to stay awake on her shift, but she soon requested a transfer to the operating room where shift rotation was not required and where night work was only necessary for emergency surgery calls. Sarah later learned that she is a "lark," or a "morning person," and also someone who is not flexible in her sleeping habits — two individual characteristics that can lead to shift work coping problems.

Another case study involves Ann, who worked as a permanent night nurse at a large metropolitan hospital. Ann was separated from her husband and trying to rear two children while earning enough money to support her family. She wanted to sleep for seven hours after her night shifts, but there was no way that she could with the demands of caring for her children and completing the household chores when she got home each morning. Ann's schedule left her little time for her friends or for uninterrupted daytime sleep. She napped in the evening before work and during her 3:00 a.m. "lunch" hour, socially isolating herself even more. Life became a seemingly unending treadmill of work, child care, and sleep. Not surprisingly, Ann's level of patient care suffered. She was desperately worried about her nursing duties, particularly right after she groggily awoke from her lunch hour nap. Ann also was concerned about her tendency to fall asleep at stop lights on the morning drive home from work. On her nights off, she reverted to sleeping at night, thus compromising her long-term adjustment to the inverted rest-activity schedule demanded by night work.

Jane's, Sarah's, and Ann's experiences illustrate some of the most common problems among nurse shift workers — sleep irregularities and social, professional, and domestic difficulties. Other common problems frequently include substance abuse, gastrointestinal disorders, and anxiety related to the biological or social stresses of shift work. Shift work is not natural to human beings. Although some people can adjust to shift work, others cannot. The nursing profession must work to accommodate those who are ill-suited for shift work, and to develop adaptation programs for those who cannot avoid it.

Summary

A considerable number of nurses are engaged in shift work due to the around-the-clock need for health care services. Although nursing organizations use a variety of shift work schedules, many have no systematic approach to shift work assignment. Nursing research has rarely focused on what is the optimum shift system for nurses and their patients.

Sleep irregularities are the most common problem for shift-working nurses, followed closely by social, professional, and domestic concerns. Shift work adaptation programs can greatly assist nurses in coping with these problems.

— Chapter 2 —

Biological Rhythms

Introduction

Most of the creatures on this planet have specific temporal, as well as spatial, niches, and the activities of individual species are best suited for particular times of the day or night. For example, owls and rats are active at night, rabbits are active at dawn and dusk, and morning larks are active in the early part of the day. As a *diurnal* species, the temporal niche of human beings is the daytime. This means that there are specific mechanisms in our physiology and anatomy that encourage us to be asleep during the nighttime and awake and active during the daytime (Arendt, Minors, and Waterhouse, 1989). This temporal specification occurs through the mechanism of a *biological clock*. The biological clock (which will be discussed in more detail later in this chapter) sends signals on a regular 24-hour basis that result in daily rhythms in almost every physiological, neuroendocrine, and psychological function that we can measure. These *circadian rhythms* serve the function of preparing human beings for restful sleep at night and active wakefulness during the day. An understanding of circadian rhythms is vital for developing appropriate shift work coping strategies.

The term *circadian*, coined by Franz Halberg in the 1950s, is derived from the Latin *circa dies*, meaning "about a day" (Halberg, 1969). The "about" part of the phrase is important, as the biological clock does not run on a precise schedule of 24.0 hours. Rather, it can be compared to a windup alarm clock, which requires periodic resetting in order to continue telling the correct time. This resetting process is a vital component of the biological clock, particularly when discussing issues related to shift work.

Although external signals are needed to keep the biological clock on track, the circadian system has a momentum of its own, and will continue to generate circadian rhythms even if the external cues of daylight or darkness are removed, if the individual stays awake all night, or (as we shall discuss in a later section) if the individual is entirely unaware of what time of day or night it is (Mills, Minors, and Waterhouse, 1978). This internal momentum of the circadian system is the most important characteristic of the biological clock when considering problems of shift work, including how nurses cope with the daily routine changes required by their work.

Although this book concentrates specifically on circadian rhythms, there are other rhythms that are equally important from a biological perspective. In fact, the discipline of chronobiology covers a whole spectrum of biological rhythms, ranging from those with periods of considerably less than a second to those with periods measured in months or even years. Short rhythms, with periods that are less than a day, are referred to as *ultradian rhythms*; rhythms with periods longer than a day are called *infradian rhythms*. The most well-known infradian rhythm is the menstrual cycle (Severino and Moline, 1989). When considered as part of the whole spectrum of biological rhythms, the menstrual cycle is clearly vulnerable when any other part of that spectrum (e.g., the circadian system) is disrupted by an abnormal work schedule. Thus, as we shall see in our discussion of health issues (Chapter 4), menstrual irregularity can be related to circadian disruptions caused by shift work.

Therefore, while we will concentrate on the circadian system in this book, it is important for the reader to understand that human chronobiology encompasses a whole spectrum of biological rhythms, and that this spectrum of rhythms comprises elements that are mutually interactive. A disruption of any one part of that spectrum can lead to a loss of harmony in many of the other parts. We will not discuss the "biorhythm" theory in this book, which postulates that several different infradian cycles are supposedly entrained at the moment of birth and remain stable throughout one's life. This theory has no reliable basis in empirical fact (U.S. Congress, 1991).

Historical Perspective

The fact that the term "circadian" was only coined in the late 1950s underscores the important point that the study of human chronobiology is a relatively new scientific discipline. In the 1950s and 1960s, most research efforts concerned simply documenting that circadian rhythms did exist, that they had a particular form, that their behavior was of a particular type, that they were predictable and nontrivial, and that they were endogenously generated (Conroy and Mills, 1970). Because of the absence of chronobiology in most medical school curricula, however, many physicians and biological scientists still only pay lip service to the concept of a biology of time and to the concept that the outcome of a particular test or a particular pharmacological intervention may be radically governed by the time of day at which it is given.

Partly because of the relative newness of the discipline of chronobiology, and partly through governmental unwillingness to prioritize research in this area, the study of human circadian rhythms has not been generously funded and the literature is thus sparse. It is important for the reader to know that there are fewer than 10 laboratories studying human circadian rhythms in the entire world, and that the total number of human subjects who have ever undergone circadian rhythms research in a controlled laboratory setting is less than 500. Therefore, the study of human circadian rhythms is not complete — much remains to be discovered. In this chapter, we will attempt to present the nurse reader with the background necessary to understand some of the circadian rhythm problems that may arise because of shift work, and will present some strategies to counter these problems.

The Biological Clock

The vast majority of experiments concerned with circadian rhythms have been conducted on rats, mice, or hamsters (Moore-Ede, Sulzman, and Fuller, 1982). These experiments usually have manipulated the light-dark cycles of rodents, and have then measured the effects of those manipulations on the animals' activity and rest patterns by counts of running wheel activity. Later experiments studied the effects of various brain lesions on the expression of circadian rhythms and on running wheel activity. For example, Rusak's (1977) classic study showed that when a particular area of the hamster brain (namely, the suprachiasmatic nuclei, or SCN — an area of the brain close to the hypothalamus) was destroyed, the normal cyclical patterns of rest and activity were disrupted. This experiment indicated that the SCN was, at the very least, an important switching station for the biological clock. Subsequent research has gone much further, showing that the SCN can generate circadian rhythms even when isolated in a petri dish, and that the SCN from one animal can be grafted onto another animal — transferring the ability to generate a coherent circadian signal. Therefore, it appears that the SCN is not only a switching station for the circadian system, it is probably the location of the biological clock itself (Moore, 1982).

One of the potential problems connected with these experiments, however, is that they were primarily conducted on nocturnal rodents, and therefore had perhaps rather questionable applicability to a diurnal species such as humans. However, careful anatomical examination has revealed that human beings also have an SCN (although, as we shall discuss later in this chapter, the question remains as to whether human beings have one circadian oscillator or two). This SCN generates most, if not all, of the observable circadian rhythms in humans.

Short-Term Time Isolation Experiments

One of the best ways to find out whether a circadian rhythm is truly endogenous (i.e., coming from the internal biological clock) is to keep a subject continuously awake in sedentary time isolation for several days. One can then be sure that any circadian rhythms that are observed are not due to either knowledge of clock time or changes in posture or waking state. This technique, referred to as the "constant conditions" protocol, was initially devised by John Mills at the University of Manchester, England (Mills, Minors, and Waterhouse, 1978), and has recently been refined by Charles Czeisler at Harvard University (Czeisler et al., 1985). Many authors have used variants of the constant conditions protocol, and Figure 2.1 presents related data that Dr. Monk collected from a laboratory group of 15 healthy young men and women. Figure 2.1 illustrates that circadian rhythms do continue to appear in both body temperature, subjective alertness (how wide awake a person feels), and objective vigilance (how well a person can detect infrequent signals). Indeed, the biological clock continues to run even when sleep is suspended and the subject is unaware of the time of day.

10

Long-Term Human Temporal Isolation Experiments

Methodology

While it is relatively easy to house a laboratory rat for several weeks in a cage that is isolated from all external time cues, it is more complicated to perform comparable experiments with human beings (some of the earliest human circadian rhythm studies were conducted in deep underground caves). When Aschoff and Wever first conducted human time isolation studies in Germany in the early-1960s, they did so in specially constructed underground bunkers that were surrounded by thick concrete walls and metal cages that provided shielding from electrical signals (Wever, 1979). For the duration of these time isolation studies, which often lasted three or four weeks, the volunteer subjects essentially were in solitary confinement.

Replacing the running wheel of the rat, the German human studies used microswitches in the floor to record the activity patterns of human subjects, as well as switches for the subjects to signal with when they went to bed and when they woke up. The most important measure, however, was body temperature, which was assessed using a rectal thermistor connected to measuring equipment via a long "umbilical cord" that the subject wore for the duration of the study. Rectal temperature has become the standard by which human circadian rhythms are assessed, for two reasons. First, rectal temperatures are easy to measure, with very little discomfort or danger occurring to the subject. Second, the rectal temperature rhythm is very stable, reliably indicating the status of the biological clock. This stability allows investigators to track the process of realignment of the biological clock in *phase-shift* experiments, where the sleep-wake cycle is abruptly changed, for example (shown later in this chapter in Figure 2.3).

Partly because of these two factors, the rectal temperature rhythm has been used to build mathematical models of the circadian system, and continues to be the measure of choice for human circadian rhythm studies. It should be noted, however, that body temperature is not the only (or most important) circadian rhythm. The neuroendocrine rhythms indicated by plasma levels of cortisol and melatonin are also vital components of the human circadian system, and would likely be the rhythms of choice if they were as easily measured as body temperature (Lewy et al., 1986; Weitzman, Czeis-

11

ler, and Moore-Ede, 1979). As we will discuss further in Chapter 8, melatonin is particularly interesting because it is only suppressed by daylight levels of illumination (Lewy et al., 1980).

When Weitzman, Czeisler, and Moore-Ede (1979) first constructed a time isolation laboratory in New York in the 1970s, it was much less extreme than Aschoff and Wever's bunker in the level of shielding subjects from external temporal signals. Weitzman's time isolation laboratory was located on the fifth floor of a busy city hospital, where blackout curtains covered the windows and air conditioning masked the outside traffic noises. Around-the-clock technicians working random-length shifts were allowed to interact with the subjects, having been carefully trained to avoid giving away time cues. In addition to the standard measures of sleep onset/ offset and rectal temperature rhythms, Weitzman's laboratory also took neuroendocrine measures from regularly obtained blood samples, and polysomnographic measures from EEG sleep tracings. This allowed the measurement of variables other than activity and body temperature, as well as the objective assessment of sleep.

Results

Despite these significant differences in experimentation methods, the overall results that were obtained from both the German and New York laboratories were very similar.

Figure 2.2 highlights data collected by Dr. Monk while working with Weitzman's group, and illustrates a very typical pattern of sleep and wakefulness that is observed when human subjects are allowed to choose their own bedtimes and waketimes in a time-isolated environment (Monk et al., 1985). This is referred to as a *free-running* experiment because the biological clock is allowed to run at its own natural period, with no constraints on that period from the outside world. The horizontal lines in Figure 2.2 represent the times during which the subject was in bed trying to sleep. Each day is plotted below the one before it. If the subject always got up and went to bed at the same clock time each day, then the horizontal bars would line up, one underneath the other. The fact that they do not, but instead drift, indicates that the natural period of this subject's biological clock was not 24 hours. By running a straight line through the sleep onset times, we find that this particular subject's biological clock period is 25.0 hours. This is precisely the pattern seen most often in both the German and New York laboratories (Weitzman, Czeisler, and Moore-Ede, 1979; Wever, 1979).

In fact, most healthy young people have free-running periods that are closer to 25 than to 24 hours, although there are differences between individuals and between men and women (with women free-running at a circadian period slightly shorter than 25 hours). Additionally, as we get older, the natural free-running period tends to shorten, so that it comes closer to 24 hours. In general, however, it remains the case that the human biological clock naturally tends to run slow, usually by up to one hour per day, which is very important when we are considering shift work implications. Because of this natural tendency to run slow, it is easier for the biological clock to accomplish *phase delays* (moving toward a later time of day) in routine than to accommodate *phase advances* (moving toward an earlier time of day). Moving routines to earlier or later times of day is, of course, an integral part of life for a nurse shift worker.

In the experiment that is illustrated in Figure 2.2, when the rhythmicity in continuously-taken rectal temperatures was measured, it was found that these temperature rhythms also ran at a period of 25 hours, similar to the sleep-wake cycle. However, for older individuals or for those experiencing very long time isolation experiments, *spontaneous internal desynchronization* can occur, which means that the temperature rhythm runs at one period (which is typically close to 25 hours), while the sleep-wake cycle runs at an entirely different period. This finding has led many researchers to believe that there is more than one circadian pacemaker in the human brain, and that one must look at multi-oscillator explanations of circadian behavior in the human being (Wever, 1975).

The practical implication of this finding for the nurse shift worker is that some oscillators may adjust to a change in schedule more slowly than others (e.g., the body temperature rhythm may take longer than the sleep-wake cycle to adjust to a run of night shifts). Studies of phase shift, either in the field as part of jet-lag-type experiments or in the laboratory as part of more rigorously controlled phase shift research, have shown that while sleep-wake cycles may appear to adjust to shift changes fairly quickly, the temperature rhythm often takes many days to adjust. By looking at the peaks and troughs of the temperature rhythm, we can measure the number of hours the rhythm is out of phase with the new shift. When we plot the number of hours out of phase as a function of consecutive days of night work, as we have in Figure 2.3, for example, we find that the adjustment rate is very slow. Indeed, even with two volunteers working 21 consecutive night shifts, it took well over a week for their biological clocks to be appropriately aligned to night work rather than day work. Aschoff et al. (1975) concluded that approximately one day of recovery was needed for each 60 minutes of phase shift being attempted in the phase advance condition, and for each 90 minutes of phase shift in the phase delay condition. A night worker typically has to phase shift his or her rhythms by at least eight hours, and often considerably more; thus, one would expect that adjustment to this changed routine would take over a week. This finding regarding the slow pace of phase shift adjustment has been proven in several field studies (e.g., Knauth et al., 1981); indeed, it has been shown that complete phase adjustment (i.e., all circadian rhythms being appropriately aligned for night work) very seldom occurs under normal circumstances.

As mentioned earlier in this chapter, the biological clock accomplishes a change in temporal orientation through the action of time cues that impinge upon the individual. These time cues are referred to as *zeitgebers*, from the German for "time giver." Zeitgebers serve two functions:

1) to keep the period of the biological clock running at exactly 24 hours, and
2) to align the biological clock to promote active wakefulness and restful sleep at the appropriate times of day and night.

Zeitgebers are particularly important when there is a major change in routine. For example, when we fly to Berlin from New York, the time cues of daylight and darkness and surrounding society all encourage our biological clock to move to an earlier time, by six hours. This process takes several days to accomplish, during which we experience symptoms of jet lag, such as sleep disruption, malaise, and gastrointestinal discomfort (Klein, Wegmann, and Hunt, 1972). In the jet lag situation, all of the zeitgebers are encouraging adjustment to the new routine. For the shift worker, however, a very different situation exists in which most of the time cues of nature and society are resolutely day-oriented, thereby slowing down any adjustment that the individual's circadian rhythms attempt to make to night work. The problem of competing zeitgebers will be addressed more fully in Chapter 8.

Just how important is it for the biological clock to be appropriately phase-adjusted? Can aberrant timings in temperature rhythms, heart rate rhythms, potassium excretion, or melatonin production really be serious enough to compromise the health, well-being, or safety of an individual shift worker? Unfortunately, the answer is yes, because the biological clock drives circadian rhythms not only in physiological variables, but also in psychological variables. These psychological variables cover a wide range, from subjective measures (such as how wide awake or content a person feels) to more objective measures of information processing, decision making, memory span, and reaction time (Colquhoun, 1971). Just as there are different circadian rhythms in body temperature and in plasma levels of cortisol and melatonin, there also are different circadian rhythms in mood, activation, and performance. These rhythms are generated by the biological clock, and therefore cannot adjust instantaneously to an abrupt change in routine, such as that caused by night work. Circadian performance rhythms are discussed in more detail in Chapter 6.

In practical terms, this means that shift-working nurses might find themselves sleepy at work in the middle of the night, and alert and unable to sleep at home during the morning hours. Additionally, memory might be impaired and manual dexterity might not be as good as at other times of day; thus, patient care could potentially suffer. In one study, for example, the long-term retention by night nurses of a training film's content was only half as good when the film was shown at 4:00 a.m. as when it was shown at 8:30 p.m (Monk and Folkard, 1978). Another sensitive measure is a process called *vigilance*, meaning a person's ability to maintain alertness in boring or nonstimulating environments. This is exactly the sort of situation that often occurs in many hospitals and nursing homes when most of the patients are asleep, but when the night nurse must be vigilant for changes in patients' conditions or activity. A study by Folkard and Monk (1979) on the time of day at which most minor hospital accidents occurred showed a circadian variation that was remarkably parallel to the circadian rhythm of vigilance found in the laboratory "constant conditions" protocol discussed earlier in this chapter (see Figure 2.4). Thus, when nurses are required to work at night during the down phase of their circadian alertness and performance cycles, the chronic jet-lag-type state that is induced can lead to malaise, irritability, and gastrointestinal distress, which can indirectly impair the nurse's ability to perform well. One must also remember that these performance decrements can be very dangerous on the nurse's drive home from work (see Chapter 8).

Individual Differences in Circadian Type

As human beings, we differ from each other in various circadian characteristics. The most obvious of these differences in circadian type is between the "morning lark," who likes to be up and about at dawn but who fades fast in the early evening, and the "night owl," who has trouble getting up in the morning but who is active and awake well into the night. When extreme morning larks are compared with extreme night owls, there are observable differences in circadian temperature and neuroendocrine rhythms (Patkai, 1971), in addition to the more obvious differences in preferred bedtimes and waketimes (Horne and Ostberg, 1976). Moreover, as we shall discuss in Chapter 7, morning larks often adjust less well to shift work than do night owls. There are other circadian type classifications concerning rigidity of sleep-wake patterns and vigor (the ability to overcome drowsiness), which are also related to shift work tolerance (Folkard, Monk, and Lobban, 1979). In discussing circadian type issues it should be noted, however, that most of us are somewhere in between extreme morning larks and extreme night owls, and for that majority one <u>can</u> make generalizations about the form and behavior of circadian rhythms.

Summary

Human beings are meant to be active during the day and to sleep at night. The internal biological clock generates circadian rhythms in physiology, activation, and performance that have a momentum of their own and are resistant to changes in routine. When adjusting to a new work/sleep routine (which often can take several days), symptoms of time lag can be experienced, sleep will be impaired, and performance may suffer.

FIGURE 2.1
Circadian Rhythms Under 36 Hours of Constant Wakeful Bedrest

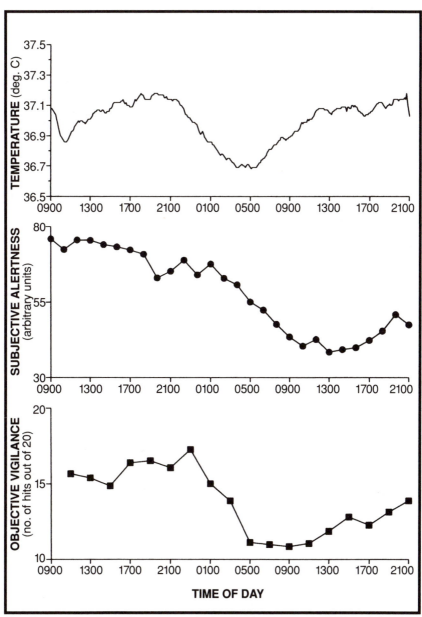

Circadian variations in rectal temperature (top), subjective alertness (middle), and objective vigilance (bottom), from a group of 15 healthy young men and women studied in a 36-hour "constant conditions" protocol.

FIGURE 2.2
Free-Running Rhythms
in a Healthy Young Man

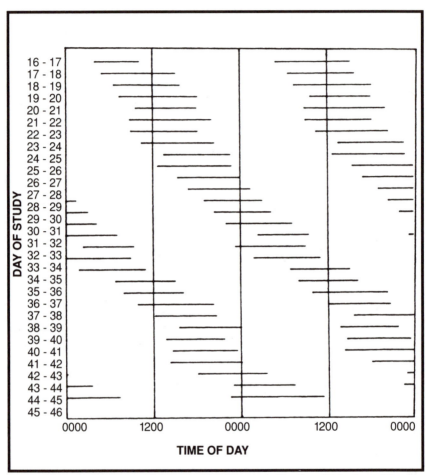

A typical free-running pattern of sleep episodes (represented by the solid horizontal lines) exhibited by a young male subject experiencing four weeks of temporal isolation. From Monk et al., 1985.

FIGURE 2.3
Pattern of Circadian Adjustment to Night Work

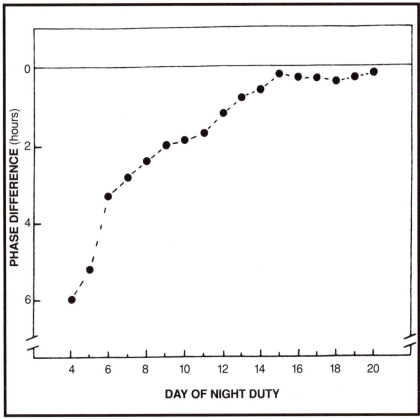

The adjustment pattern of the circadian temperature rhythm phase of two young male subjects experiencing 21 consecutive night shifts. The horizontal line at zero represents a perfect nocturnal orientation. From Folkard and Monk, 1979.

FIGURE 2.4
Laboratory Vigilance and Minor Hospital Accidents

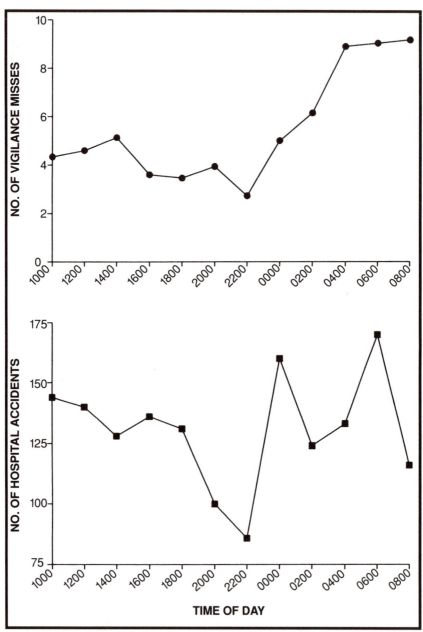

Circadian variation in objective vigilance from the laboratory (*N*=15) [top], and a count of minor hospital accidents over a five-year period [bottom]. In both cases, increases on the y-axis represent *worsening* performance. From Folkard, Monk, and Lobban, 1978.

Chapter 3

Social, Professional, and Domestic Issues

Introduction

Almost every aspect of our society is structured to encourage people to work during the day and to relax in the evening and on weekends. Life can be difficult for those whose schedules do not fit this routine. For instance, imagine how day workers would complain if the television repairman would only come "sometime between midnight and 6:00 a.m.," if all deliveries were made during the middle of the night, and if the telephone rang incessantly during these hours. For night nurses, this scenario is a reality: every facet of society seems to intrude while they are attempting to sleep.

However, it is not just the world outside the shift worker's home that is noisy and demanding during the day — often, the home itself is also at its noisiest. In shared apartments, for instance, roommates come and go, often working diverse schedules. For parents working evening or night shifts, children may be getting ready for school in the morning, playing in the house during the day, or requiring help with schoolwork in the evening. Additionally, housework and laundry need to be done, and the telephone frequently rings. All of these demands and interruptions to the shift worker's sleeptime can lead to tensions within the family. These social and domestic problems often spill over into the nurse's professional life, creating further problems in the workplace.

While sleep is the problem mentioned most frequently by shift workers, social and domestic problems also are top concerns. Shift work forces nurses to make basic changes in the way they allocate time to social, professional, and domestic activities, all of which are disrupted by a work schedule that usually limits interactions with family, friends, and colleagues. Chapter 1 introduced the case of Ann, who was having trouble rearing two children and performing effectively as a full-time night shift nurse. Her case illustrates some of the social, professional, and domestic problems connected with the pressures and demands placed on a nurse shift worker by family and society. This chapter focuses on disturbances in the nurse's roles as an involved member of society and the nursing profession, a spouse, and/or a parent, summarizing some of the relevant research findings on this topic. As is true of so much of the research in this field, however, subjects were often European male industrial shift workers, although there have been studies of nurses as well.

Social and Professional Roles

Nurse shift workers must function in a society largely organized around daytime, weekday work schedules. Within this environment, different social concerns exist for the evening shift nurse, the night shift nurse, and the rotating shift nurse.

Although individual schedules, interests, life-styles, and habits all have an impact on one's social life, there is some general agreement on the social effects of shift work. For instance, shift workers are not as likely as day workers to join political, civic, recreational, or professional organizations, to attend meetings, or to hold offices (Walker, 1985). Nurse shift workers usually find it easier to maintain informal contact with friends through telephone calls or casual get-togethers than to attend regularly scheduled family and social events (Skipper, Jung, and Coffey, 1990). For solitary hobbies and activities such as gardening and housework, however, shift work may be an advantage, A large study of Dutch nurses found that, in general, shift work takes a greater toll on the social well-being of married nurses than on their unmarried colleagues because of the greater obligations married nurses have to their families (Bosch and de Lange, 1987). This study also found that 70% of these nurse shift workers saw family and friends less than when they worked days.

The Evening Shift

Although working the evening shift on a permanent or rotating basis does not disrupt, to any great extent, normal biological circadian rhythms, sleep-wake cycles, or eating patterns, it does have major effects on many nurses' social and professional relationships. When working the evening shift, for example, nurses frequently have to decline social invitations and miss professional meetings. A study of 463 nurses found that evening shift nurses participated the least often in voluntary organizations (day shift nurses participated the most frequently, followed by night shift nurses, and then rotating shift nurses) [Skipper, Jung, and Coffey, 1990]. Evening shift nurses also were found to spend the greatest amount of time in solitary activities.

On the positive side, however, evening shift nurses have more time for shopping and errands, lunching with friends, gardening, sports, and housework. Additionally, evening shift nurses generally have the potential to sleep longer than day or night nurses.

The Night Shift

In contrast to evening shift nurses, many night shift nurses do not get enough sleep and may suffer from desynchrony of their physiological circadian rhythms. Although many complain of being chronically sleep deprived, night shift nurses are able to participate in some daytime and early evening social and professional activities. Nurses enrolled in academic programs, for instance, often request fixed night shifts in order to avoid shift rotation and to accommodate class schedules. In a large National Institute of Occupational Safety and Health (NIOSH) study of RNs and LPNs from 12 U.S. hospitals, permanent night shift nurses were more satisfied than evening or rotating shift nurses with the time available for social activities, sports, errands, personal activities, and child care (Tasto and Colligan, 1978). A small study of English nurses speculates that permanent night shift nurses who are introverts, with few social activities and rigid schedules, adapt more easily to night work (Adams, Folkard, and Young, 1986).

Rotating Shifts

For nurses working rotating shifts, it is their variable schedule that interferes with social and professional activities. Involvement in any activity requiring regular attendance may be nearly impossible unless nurses know their schedules well in advance. If they cannot predict their hours of work, rotating shift nurses may hesitate to commit themselves to activities such as PTA meetings, community board meetings, committee work for their district nurses association, or a continuing education program. Researchers have found that rotating shift workers get less sleep than permanent shift workers, and may lack a feeling of well-being and the energy to use their free time for social or professional activities (Colligan and Rosa, 1990). In a large U.S. study, Gordon et al. (1986) found that women who worked rotating shifts scored lower on a measure of social networking than those on fixed shifts.

Moonlighting

Moonlighting is a work issue often associated with shift workers (Mott et al., 1965). Some European studies of "double jobbing," as it is also called, have shown that this practice is more common among shift workers than day workers (Walker, 1985). Ample opportunities for secondary nursing positions exist for nurse shift workers through temporary staffing agencies and the health care institutions themselves. In fact, the 1988 National Sample Survey of Registered Nurses estimated that 13.8% of all employed nurses held secondary nursing positions (Moses, 1990). For one-third of these, the moonlighting position involved hospital staff nurse work. Unfortunately, we do not know how many of these moonlighters were shift workers in their primary or secondary positions. Without empirical data, we cannot be certain that more North American nurse shift workers hold secondary positions than do day-working shift nurses. It is likely, however, that nurses working 12-hour shifts (only three times per week, on average) engage in moonlighting more frequently than those on eight-hour schedules. For nurses who are already sleep-deprived and fatigued, however, the added exhaustion of moonlighting can increase the risks of practice errors or of accidents on the drive home.

Ninety-six percent of RNs are women, and since women in our society are often homemakers in addition to working outside the home, a moonlighting position actually may be the nurse's third job. While secondary nursing positions are often relatively easy to find and to vacate, the nurse is often too dependent on the additional income to make use of this flexibility and to abandon the secondary position when other problems arise. Although two work commitments outside the home might be manageable until children come along, an elderly relative needs care, or the after-school baby-sitter quits, each additional commitment increases the shift worker's level of stress — stress that inevitably will diminish the nurse shift worker's quality of nursing care and job satisfaction.

Domestic Roles

The home life of the nurse shift worker is a potential source of both support and stress. The majority of registered nurses are married and have children at home. In 1988, it was estimated that over 70% of RNs were married, 55% had children at home, and 21.5% had children under the age of six (Moses, 1990). Four domestic roles concern us in regard to the nurse shift worker:

- homemaker,
- sexual partner,
- social companion, and
- parent.

All of these roles are complex and require much further study in order to develop coping strategies to benefit nurse shift workers and those living in their households.

Homemaker

All aspects of homemaking do not suffer equally because of a shift work assignment. One large U.S. study confirmed that rotating and fixed evening and night shift workers spent four to six hours more each week on housework than did day shift workers. Day shift nurses may use less free time for housework and more for social and professional activities, an option less available to the evening shift nurse. The researchers' tentative explanation for this finding is that some shift workers sleep less than day workers, and that housework is a domestic task that can be performed at any time of the day or night (with some exceptions, of course). The investigators also found more conflict between work and domestic life for shift workers because of scheduling difficulties with their families. The time that the shift worker has available for other domestic activities often occurs at the wrong time of day for the rest of the household (Staines and Pleck, 1984). Cooking dinner for a spouse who works days, when the night nurse would rather be cooking breakfast, is an example of the type of homemaking problem that must be resolved. Additionally, as mentioned earlier, night nurses frequently encounter the problem of repair and delivery persons stopping by the house while they attempt to sleep.

Sexual Partner

Sex is frequently mentioned as a problem by shift workers when they discuss social and domestic issues. The day worker's routine of work, recreation, and sleep is more conducive to a satisfactory sex life than the night worker's pattern of work, sleep, and recreation. Following the relaxation of an evening's recreation together, two day shift workers can retire to bed; not so for night nurses who have to report to work. Time for intimacy is one more problem to solve. In the large NIOSH study, fixed night shift workers were the least satisfied with their sexual activities, followed by rotating shift workers (Tasto and Colligan, 1978).

Social Companion

Solving companionship problems can be difficult for partners who work different shifts. Some experts attribute the high divorce rate experienced by shift workers to spouses who dislike staying home alone in the evening or at night and react by separating (U.S. Congress, 1991). Other investigators caution that the survey research on family and social relations does not allow us, for example, to "determine whether rotating shift work causes marital dissatisfaction, or whether unhappily married people choose rotating shifts to escape domestic strife" (Colligan and Rosa, 1990, p. 316).

Parent

The problems of shift workers who are parents of children living at home have been studied somewhat more frequently than other facets of the shift worker's domestic role. Perhaps this is because of the high incidence of parents who also are shift workers. In studying a national cohort of the U.S. population, Presser (1987) found that shift work was more common among young workers than older ones, and among parents than childless workers.

We know that permanent night work is selected by some nurses so that they can be at home with their children during the day or evening hours (Alward, 1986). Particularly for nurses who face the alternative of rotating shifts, child care may be easier to provide when working a fixed night shift. In the NIOSH study, permanent night shift nurses were found to be more satisfied than permanent evening or rotating shift workers with the time available for child care (Tasto and Colligan, 1978). However, the time allocated for parenting activities often comes at the expense of the shift worker's sleep. A study of the sleep habits of French nursing personnel working fixed night shifts found that unmarried female nurses without children averaged well over an hour a day more sleep than the married mothers of two children (Gadbois, 1981). Eighty-five percent of the 898 night nursing personnel surveyed in this study requested the night shift, most frequently citing family responsibilities as the reason for their choice. Female night shift nurses with children at home clearly gave priority to family responsibilities over daytime sleep.

Although nurses working 12-hour shifts might have to leave for work at 6:00 p.m., or might not get home until 8:00 p.m., they do have more days off each week, and, therefore, have the potential to spend more time with their children than permanent evening shift nurses.

The evening shift can be disastrous for the parenting role. Much interaction with school-age children occurs between 4:00 and 9:00 p.m., precisely when the evening shift nurse is working. Schools operate under the assumption that children will be at school while their parents are at work, and teacher conferences, PTA meetings, and school board meetings are usually held in the evening.

Summary

Competing social, professional, and domestic demands add stress to the lives of nurse shift workers of both sexes. Concerns about these demands are reported by shift workers almost as frequently as sleep disorders, and are just as important as biological concerns. Nurse shift workers must pay attention to social, professional, and domestic issues, or they will not cope well with shift work.

— Chapter 4 —

Health Issues

Introduction

As we have detailed in earlier chapters, shift work is inherently unnatural to human beings. *Homo sapiens* is a diurnal species endowed with a physiology based on the premise that activity will take place primarily during the day, that sleep will occur primarily at night, and that these two states will cycle on a regular schedule.

Human beings frequently engage in many other activities, however, that also are essentially unnatural without necessarily being harmful. For instance, flying in airplanes and living in air-conditioned buildings are basically unnatural activities, but they are not considered high-risk by most of us. Similarly, shift work does not necessarily have to be a high-risk activity.

Nurse shift workers must determine whether they have a decreased sense of well-being and an increased risk of stress, illness, or early death related to their hours of work. A major premise of this book is that, while they may be at some degree of health risk due to the nature of their work schedules, nurse shift workers can minimize any risks to themselves and to their patients, clients, colleagues, and communities by learning and incorporating shift work coping techniques.

Research interest in the health of shift workers has grown throughout the 20th century. Beginning in Europe and spreading to much of the industrialized world, researchers have increasingly

29

investigated the relationships of well-being and illness to shift work. Much of this research has focused on European males working in manufacturing settings. Since the early 1970s, however, there has been increased interest in both male and female shift workers in the service sector.

Researchers have found that the biggest differences in health do not occur between shift workers and day workers, but between former shift workers and day workers. Not unexpectedly, those individuals who gave up shift work because they could not cope well with it reported more health problems than those who continued with shift work. Several studies report that up to 20% of all shift workers are unable to cope with working night or rotating shifts (Rutenfranz et al., 1977). Another finding generally supported throughout the literature is that both rotating and night shift workers have more health complaints than either day or evening shift workers. Rotating shift workers report the highest number of physical and psychological symptoms, though it is not always clear in these cases whether morbidity developed independently or was related to shift work (Scott and LaDou, 1990). The reader should bear in mind that, while many shift workers are not coping well with their work schedules and do experience a decrease in well-being, causal relationships have rarely been definitively established. Reasons for this are discussed later in this chapter.

Stress and Strain Concept

In a review of occupational health problems related to shift work, Rutenfranz (1982) describes his "stress and strain" concept, which suggests that stresses related to the phase shifts of sleeping and waking hours in some shift workers can lead to strain that may eventually affect the well-being, health, performance, and social lives of these workers. However, there are many intervening variables that influence how much and what type of strain an individual shift worker might experience and what form it will take.

Rutenfranz's model includes three groups of variables that can affect shift work strain:

Personal Variables
- age,
- circadian type,
- personality, and
- physiological adaptability;

Work Variables
- type of work,
- length of shift,
- shift system and schedule,
- relationships with colleagues, and
- work environment;

Social and Domestic Variables
- marital status,
- number of dependents,
- housing conditions, and
- community relationships.

In addition to these three groups of variables, an individual's level of commitment to shift work and the self-selection at play in shift worker samples help explain why research into the risks and health consequences of shift work often reaches conflicting results. For obvious reasons, one rarely sees random sampling used for assignment to different shift work groups in these studies; subjects are already in the various shift system groupings. The level of commitment by shift workers to their hours of work is exhibited by the degree to which they adjust their social schedules, sleeptimes, physical activities, and dietary habits.

By applying knowledge of coping strategies that decrease the stress of shift work and thus facilitate adaptation (discussed in Chapter 8), shift workers and their employers can diminish the adverse impact of shift work on health. It is important that shift workers do not convince themselves that health disorders are unavoidable as a result of shift work, or that their lives inevitably will be shortened. Although reduced life spans do occur in some laboratory animals put on mock rotating shift schedules, this finding is contradicted by studies with other animals that show lengthened life spans. Most importantly, there currently is no evidence for reduced life spans in shift-working humans. The fact remains, however, that many shift workers may experience adverse health consequences as a result of not coping well with shift work schedules. This chapter focuses on those potential health problems of particular concern for the nurse shift worker.

31

The Health of Nurse Shift Workers

A fairly extensive body of research literature describes the relationships between health and shift work, although long-term studies are rare because they are methodologically difficult to carry out. As we pointed out earlier, many of the subjects are European males from industrial settings. Female shift workers are, however, receiving an increased amount of attention.

Sleep and digestive system disorders are the health deficits most often associated with rotating and permanent night shift work. Psychological problems are also evident, to a lesser degree. In a large U.S. study of the impact of shift work on health behaviors, social network participation, and perceived stress, rotating shift workers fared worse than fixed shift workers (Gordon et al., 1986). Unfortunately, permanent night shift workers were not separated from permanent day and evening shift workers in this study. After controlling for differences in age, income, and education, individuals who rotated between day and night shifts reported significantly more job stress and emotional problems than did permanent shift workers. Female rotating shift workers consistently had lower social network scores, drank more alcohol, and took more sleeping pills and tranquilizers than did female permanent shift workers. Male rotating shift workers used more digestive aids than did their fixed shift counterparts; this difference was not found between the female rotating and fixed shift groups. There were no significant differences among the rotating and fixed shift groups in levels of cigarette smoking or caffeine ingestion.

The literature dealing specifically with the stresses and health deficits of nurse shift workers describes similar findings. In a study of over 400 registered nurses working in five Southeastern U.S. hospitals, researchers found a strong relationship between shift work and job-related stress (Coffey, Skipper, and Jung, 1988). Rotating shift nurses experienced the most job-related stress, followed by evening, day, and night shift nurses. The researchers suggest that rotating shift nurses suffer from disturbed circadian rhythms and a lack of consistency in collegial relationships, while most permanent night shift nurses work at a slower pace and have less opportunities than other shift-working nurses for interpersonal conflict with staff and patients. The researchers concluded that in health care facilities where the work environment and the division of labor vary by shift, it is difficult to differentiate the effects of stress caused by circadian rhythm disruption from those caused by the work itself.

In a recent report on the implications of biological rhythms for the worker (U.S. Congress, 1991), 15 studies on the health consequences of shift work for nurses are highlighted, including five that investigated the health of North American nurses. Twelve of the 15 studies reported sleep disturbances and deficits among the rotating and permanent night shift nurse subjects. Our own interviews of night shift nurses confirm that the quality and quantity of sleep obtained are often the main factors in determining how long a nurse remains on permanent night shifts or tolerates shift rotation. In Chapter 1, sleep was a problem for the three nurses described; each suffered a decrease in well-being related to sleep deficits. (Sleep is the subject of Chapter 5, and sleep management is discussed in Chapters 7 and 8.)

Gastrointestinal Disorders

In addition to sleep problems, nurse shift workers may encounter a variety of other health disturbances, such as problems with their gastrointestinal systems. Such disorders are frequently mentioned by night shift nurses, and night work was cited as the cause of weight problems and poor eating habits by many of the nurses we interviewed for this book. Many hospitals and health care facilities do not provide hot meal services in a normal social environment during the night shift, although microwave ovens are generally available for heating food brought from home or purchased from vending machines.

After controlling for age and marital status, rotating shift nurses in the NIOSH study reported significantly more digestive problems than three fixed shift groups, and ate more snack foods (Tasto and Colligan, 1978). Permanent night shift nurses reported eating fewer meals in a 24-hour period than the other groups. In a Belgian study, rotating night shift nurses reported significantly higher levels of indigestion and disrupted appetites than did their permanent night shift counterparts (Verhaegen et al., 1987). A Finnish study of nurses and nursing assistants working rotating shifts in one hospital also found that married workers reported more gastrointestinal symptoms (such as poor appetite, distention, constipation, and diarrhea) than did single workers (Harma, Ilmarinen, and Knauth, 1988). A possible explanation for this finding might be that married nurse shift workers make special efforts to stick with their families' diurnal eating schedules, even when such efforts interfere with sleep patterns, biological rhythms, and energy levels.

Night work is thought by some authorities to be a minor risk factor in the development of duodenal ulcers (Rutenfranz, Haider, and Koller, 1985). As with other types of health problems, peptic ulcer disease has been found to occur significantly more frequently among day workers who left shift work than among those who had never worked rotating or night shifts (Scott and LaDou, 1990). It is logical that a disruption in the normal circadian rhythms of gastrointestinal enzyme secretion would affect digestion and diseases of the gastrointestinal system. Even in light of new research linking gastritis and ulcers with the H. pylori bacterium (Dyer, 1993), we conclude that the stress of night work and its attendant diet and digestive problems may aggravate ulcer disease.

Cardiovascular Disorders

The links between shift work and cardiovascular disease are less conclusive than those between shift work and gastrointestinal problems. Most lists of cardiovascular risk factors include elevated low-density lipoprotein and serum cholesterol, hypertension, smoking, obesity, and a sedentary life-style. Shift work is farther down on such lists because the association between shift work and cardiovascular disease has been studied less.

We think it is safe to assume that rotating shift work in particular contributes at least a degree of risk of heart disease, perhaps in relationship to the stress it causes some individuals. An example of the type of study that led to our conclusion is a 15-year follow-up study of Swedish male paper mill workers (Knutsson et al., 1986). The investigators found an increased risk of ischemic heart disease (IHD) in rotating shift workers, after controlling for age and smoking habits. Regression analysis showed that age was the main predictor of IHD, followed by shift work. In another study, after controlling for smoking habits, obesity, diet, and physical activity, the investigators found a significant association between irregular work hours and higher total and low-density lipoprotein cholesterol and lower high-density lipoprotein cholesterol (DeBacker et al., 1984).

We could find little in the literature that included female shift workers in studies of cardiovascular disease and shift work. None of the nurses we interviewed complained of problems related to the cardiovascular system. The NIOSH study, however, reported that, after controlling for age and marital status, rotating shift nurses had a significantly higher incidence of chest pains and pressures than did fixed evening or night shift nurses (Tasto and Colligan, 1978).

Menstruation and Pregnancy Disorders

Because 96% of the nurses in the United States are women, we summarize here the little and often conflicting data concerning the effects of shift work on menstruation and childbearing. The NIOSH study reported that rotating shift nurses had significantly longer menstrual periods and suffered more accompanying sickness, weakness, nervousness, and tension than fixed shift nurses (Tasto and Colligan, 1978). Both fixed night and rotating shift nurses spent more time lying down due to menstrual cramps than did evening nurses, and night shift nurses also spent more time lying down than did day shift nurses. These findings were not consistent for the food processor sample in the same study. For example, rotating shift food processors felt less tense and nervous when menstruating than did fixed shift food processors. Food processors who worked rotating and night shifts experienced significantly more irregular menstrual periods than did the fixed day and afternoon shift groups. In contrast, night and rotating shift nurses had significantly fewer irregular menstrual periods than day shift nurses. Another investigator who studied 146 RNs from one U.S. hospital found no differences between fixed and rotating shift nurses in menstrual flow, incidence of dysmenorrhea, or other menstrual characteristics (Kuchinski, 1989).

Menstruation and pregnancy disorders related to shift work also have been studied in Japan. In a large study that included 946 nurses and 876 other women, participants who worked rotating night shifts reported higher rates of menstrual irregularity and painful menstruation than did those who worked fixed day shifts (Uehata and Sasakawa, 1982). When day and rotating shift workers of childbearing ages were compared, the day shift workers had a significantly higher rate of pregnancies and deliveries, while the rotating shift workers had a higher rate of abortions. There were no significant differences between the two groups in the rate of abnormal deliveries.

The correlation between shift work and fatigue has been implicated as a risk factor for premature birth. In a survey of 3,437 women, researchers found a significantly increased risk of premature birth related to shift work fatigue (Mamalle, Lauman, and Lazar, 1984). A significant relationship also was found between premature births and high fatigue scores on an index that included elements of physical exertion, mental stress, environmental conditions (noise, heat, cold, chemicals), standing, and working on machines. Working over 41 hours per week was associated with more premature births than part-time work or a 40-hour work week. There was a combined effect of working more than 40 hours per week and occupational fatigue. In the Uehata and Sasakawa (1982) study, women working rotating night shifts reported significantly more fatigue symptoms (including general fatigue, depressed vitality, anxiety, irritability, and physical disorders) than did female day shift workers. In some of the occupational sections of a sample of 22,761 women, Canadian investigators found strong associations between rotating shift work and premature births, and between rotating shift work and low birth weights (McDonald et al., 1988).

More data were available on the relationships between rotating shift work and pregnancy than between permanent night shift work and pregnancy. In view of the sleep deficits and fatigue reported by nurse shift workers and other occupational groups of women, as well as the nurse's potential for strenuous work and mental stress, rotating shift work should be considered an additional stressor for the pregnant nurse. When possible, overtime should also be avoided (Scott and LaDou, 1990).

Psychological Disorders

It is important to point out that the substantial body of research concerning the relationship between shift work and psychological disorders supports an <u>association</u> between the two conditions, but does not provide firm evidence of cause-and-effect, due to methodological problems. These methodological problems include the intervening variables discussed earlier in this chapter, such as self-selection in group assignment and the lack of longitudinal studies.

In this book, we have attempted to establish a strong relationship between shift work and circadian system disruption, and between shift work and a variety of physiological, psychological, and social stressors. These factors are also suspected of being associated with psychiatric disorders such as depression, neuroses, and substance abuse. Much of the current research on the human biological clock is being conducted within psychiatry departments because of the important link that has been established between disorders of the biological clock and depression. Psychiatrists once hoped that some types of depression could be relieved through changes in the patient's sleep-wake cycle. Although that hope has not been realized, we do know that depression leads to disorders of the biological clock (Wehr and Goodwin, 1983). There is certainly a risk that the converse also may be true.

In the NIOSH study, nurses' psychological states were measured using the Profile of Mood States (POMS) [Tasto and Colligan, 1978]. On the POMS subscales, rotating shift nurses exhibited significantly more feelings of depression and dejection than either fixed day or night shift nurses, and more feelings of tension and anxiety than either fixed evening or night shift nurses. The rotating shift nurses also reported significantly less vigor and more fatigue, more confusion, and more bewilderment than all fixed shift nurse groups. Personality traits of the nurse sample were measured on the Eysenck Personality Inventory (EPI). Rotating shift nurses scored significantly higher on neuroticism and significantly lower on sociability than did any of the fixed shift groups, while evening and night shift nurses scored significantly higher on sociability than day shift nurses.

The EPI also was used to assess the shift work tolerance of 128 Finnish rotating shift nurses and nursing assistants (Harma, Ilmarinen, and Knauth, 1988). The more neurotic nurses (as measured by the EPI) were more likely to report gastrointestinal symptoms and fatigue. A Canadian study also found that rotating shift nurses had significantly higher scores on a depression scale and significantly lower scores on a physical health scale than did a mixed group of permanent shift nurses (Jamal and Jamal, 1982).

In a large study of French female hospital workers, sleep impairment was the only mental health indicator that was significantly different for groups of day, evening, and night shift nurses (Estryn-Behar et al., 1990). Night shift nurses reported more sleep impairment than the other groups, but not more fatigue or use of drugs, and no less mental well-being. (Rotating shift workers were not mentioned in this report.)

In general, when compared to permanent day shift workers, rotating shift and permanent night and evening shift workers have higher rates of substance abuse (Cole, Loving, and Kripke, 1990). Rather surprisingly, we could find little in the literature specific to shift work and substance abuse by nurses. The NIOSH study did examine the use of alcohol and medications by nurses and food processors, including stimulants and depressants (Tasto and Colligan, 1978). Rotating and evening shift nurses reported drinking significantly more beer than day nurses. Rotating shift nurses consumed more liquor of all types than did night shift nurses. Fixed night shift nurses reported drinking fewer days each week but drinking before work more often than any other shift group. The use of stimulants was significantly higher among rotating shift nurses only when compared to evening shift nurses. No significant differences were found among the groups of nurses in the use of hypnotics; however, in the food processor groups, the rotating shift workers took sleeping medications significantly more often than the three fixed shift groups. Since the use of self-reported data to study alcohol and medication abuse is subject to response bias, it would be enlightening to study the relationship between shift work and substance abuse among those nurses who seek treatment for their addictions.

Not all studies, however, support a significant relationship between shift work and nurses' mental and physical health. The researchers who found a significant relationship between shift work and job-related stress did not find significant correlations between shift work and the nurses' physical health (Coffey, Skipper, and Jung, 1988), nor between shift work and mental depression when the means were adjusted for background variables such as age and the desire to change shifts (Skipper, Jung, and Coffey, 1990). These investigators conjecture that the unexpected findings may be related to each shift's different work requirements, the self-selection involved in shift work assignments, and the varied reasons nurses have for making a commitment to shift work. These findings illustrate the complexity of shift work research and the need to control intervening variables, including the influence of each shift's different tasks and requirements. To reiterate an earlier point, perhaps we need to study the health effects of shift work on nurses who leave shift work rather than those committed to permanent or rotating shift work schedules.

Shift Maladaptation Syndrome

Most nurses beginning night shift work, whether on a fixed or rotating basis, will experience some symptoms of circadian rhythm disruption. The majority of these nurses eventually will adapt to shift work, at least to the extent that deficits in their well-being are not severe. The NIOSH study concluded that the workers who adapted best to shift work were those who had more positive attitudes toward their jobs, shift hours, and coworkers; who had spouses who complained less about their shift-working schedules;

who were less neurotic, more impulsive, and more extroverted; and who used less medications, but more frequently used alcohol to enhance sleep (Tasto and Colligan, 1978).

Shift workers who do not cope well with their schedules (up to 20% of all shift workers) have been described as suffering from *shift maladaptation syndrome* (SMS) [Moore-Ede and Richardson, 1985]. These shift workers never adjust to their hours of work, or their adjustment deteriorates as they age. Several characteristics of SMS, as summarized from Scott and LaDou (1990), include the following:

- sleep disturbances and chronic tiredness;
- gastrointestinal complaints, such as heartburn, constipation, and diarrhea;
- alcohol or drug abuse (usually related to self-treatment of insomnia);
- higher rates of accidents or near-misses;
- depression, fatigue, mood disturbances, malaise, or personality changes; and/or
- difficulties with interpersonal relationships.

Risk factors for SMS include being over 40 years old, living with persons who have regular daytime schedules, and a poor tolerance of circadian rhythm disruptions (as evidenced after air travel and daylight-savings time changes, for example).

Although other causes of SMS symptoms must first be ruled out, it is the history of shift work and the combination of symptoms that often lead to a diagnosis of SMS. Nurses should consider the possibility of SMS when assessing the health of clients, as well as their own health. Scott and LaDou (1990) state that the only effective treatment for SMS involves removing the nurse from shift work. It is our opinion, however, that much can be done to help the nurse cope with shift work before taking that final step. Assessing the nurse's desire to adapt to shift work is an essential first step. As we concluded in our own comparative study of rotating and permanent night shift nurses, differences between the two groups' levels of commitment to shift work, life-styles, and home environments appeared more likely to account for the permanent shift nurses' higher ratings of subjective well-being than any differences in biological rhythm adjustment (Alward and Monk, 1990).

Medical Contraindications for Shift Work

As described in Chapter 2, almost every physiological function that can be measured in humans follows a circadian rhythm — demonstrating a high and low value once in each 24-hour period when synchronized to the environment. Chronopharmacologists have studied the influences of biological rhythms on medications, as well as the effects of medications on the biological clock (Smolensky and Reinberg, 1990). The desynchronization of circadian rhythms and the sleep deficits that are associated with shift work have been found to have harmful effects on some existing health disorders and their pharmacological treatments (Scott and LaDou, 1990). Much more attention should be given to these findings by the health professions in light of the increasing number of shift workers within their own ranks and among their clientele.

Scott and LaDou (1990) provide a summary of the definite medical contraindications for shift work, which include the following:

- epilepsy requiring medication within the last year;
- coronary artery disease, especially if there is unstable angina or a history of myocardial infarction;
- asthma requiring regular medication, especially if the patient is steroid-dependent;
- insulin-dependent diabetes mellitus (IDDM) [Workers with IDDM may be able to tolerate a permanent night shift if regularity in meals, activity, and medication can be maintained during work days and days off.];
- hypertension requiring multiple drugs;
- polypharmacy in general if there are circadian variations in the effectiveness of any medication, especially if a rotating schedule is being considered;
- recurrent peptic ulcer disease;
- irritable bowel syndrome, if symptoms are severe;
- chronic depression or other psychiatric disorder requiring medication; and/or
- a history of shift maladaptation syndrome .

Some of the existing medical disorders identified by Scott and LaDou (1990) as relative contraindications for shift work include:

- mild asthma;
- non-insulin-dependent diabetes mellitus;
- a history of depression;

- a history of seizures, but not currently requiring medication and no seizures for at least one year;
- mild irritable bowel syndrome;
- Crohn's disease;
- frequent indigestion;
- insomnia;
- cardiac risk factors, such as elevated serum cholesterol or hypertension, particularly in conjunction with cigarette smoking or a family history of coronary artery disease; and/or
- use of a medication known to have significant time-of-day variations in effectiveness.

Both definite and relative contraindications for shift work should be used for counseling prospective employees, and for monitoring the occupational health of current shift-working nurses. Individual characteristics, such as level of commitment to shift work, age, and circadian type, play an important role in determining whether nurses and their clients should undertake shift work in the presence of any of the conditions described above. Nurses should make informed decisions about their personal abilities to cope with shift work. Additionally, it is essential for nurse managers to assess employees' levels of commitment to shift work, and to listen to prospective or current shift workers' evaluations of their ability to adapt to particular hours of work in light of individual physical, psychological, and social risk factors. (Shift work assessment strategies and techniques are presented in Chapter 7).

Summary

In this chapter, we have highlighted a variety of health disorders that are often associated with shift work, and have found convincing support for a "stress and strain" concept of shift work (Rutenfranz, 1982). When stresses do develop, the resulting strain can adversely affect the health of the shift worker. Although shift-working nurses complain more of sleep and gastrointestinal disorders than of cardiovascular, reproductive, or psychological concerns, all of these health deficits may occur. Our aim in this book is to help nurse shift workers develop assessment and coping strategies, rather than to simply brace themselves for impaired health and well-being.

— Chapter 5 —

Sleep Issues

Introduction

A common misperception of sleep is that it is merely a state of blissful oblivion — comparable to a television set when it is switched off, and hardly worthy of serious study. Nothing, however, could be further from the truth. Sleep is an active process that is not uniform throughout the night, but which can be characterized into different types and depths (Mendelson, 1987).

This realization about the nature of sleep is relatively recent. Up until the mid-1950s (with the exception of dream content interpretation), scientists and physicians largely ignored sleep as an object of study. This oversight changed as a result of the work of Nathaniel Kleitman at the University of Chicago, who first objectively recorded sleep using the polygraph (Aserinsky and Kleitman, 1953; Dement and Kleitman, 1957). In doing so, Kleitman and his students discovered the true heterogeneous nature of sleep, and laid the foundation for the whole discipline of sleep research and sleep disorders medicine (which is now an active discipline with its own academic society and journals). Currently, there are more than 100 sleep disorders clinics across the country, and several government initiatives supporting sleep research and sleep disorders medicine.

How Sleep Is Measured

The main mechanisms by which sleep is measured are the amplification and recording of the minute electrical impulses representing the electroencephalogram (EEG), the electrooculogram (EOG), and the electromyogram (EMG). Unlike the standard EEG evaluation, sleep EEG evaluations last the whole night and involve a small number of electrodes. Typically, in addition to the ground and reference electrodes, two electrodes (in the C3 and C4 positions on the top of the head) are used to monitor the EEG signal (which measures brain wave activity), two electrodes near the temples are used to measure the eye movement (EOG) signal, and two electrodes are used on the chin to measure muscle tone (EMG). These signals are amplified and traced throughout the night using either the paper trace of a polygraph or an electronic analogue of it. At the end of a night of recording, there typically are about 1,000 feet of paper trace to be scored (see Figure 5.1). To make the scoring task more manageable, the sleep record is divided into one-minute or 30-second epochs, and each epoch is categorized individually (Rechtschaffen and Kales, 1968).

Sleep Types and Stages

Expert sleep scorers view the overall pattern of EEG, EOG, and EMG traces for a particular epoch, and categorize the epoch into one of two types of sleep: REM (rapid eye movement) or non-REM. Although rapid eye movements are the most obvious marker for REM sleep, there are others — namely, a drop-off in EMG signals (i.e., a loss of muscle tone) and an "almost awake" EEG pattern. When awakened from REM sleep, individuals typically report being in the middle of a narrative-style dream. Although dreaming can occur in other sleep stages, and REM sleep is not <u>always</u> associated with dreaming, it is not inaccurate to refer to REM sleep as "dream sleep." When deprived of REM sleep, enough "pressure" (need for REM sleep) builds up for the individual to rapidly enter an "REM rebound," where above-normal levels of REM sleep and reported dreaming occur for one or two nights. Early reports of psychoses being induced by REM deprivation, however, appear to have been exaggerated (Horne, 1988).

If a sleep epoch is categorized as non-REM, the EEG signal is further examined to categorize the epoch into one of four possible sleep stages, with stage 1 being the lightest sleep and stage 4 being the deepest sleep. Stages 3 and 4 are collectively referred to as slow wave sleep (SWS), or "delta" sleep, because of the delta waves mapped out by the EEG trace. SWS is the first sleep stage to be recovered after sleep deprivation, and appears to be the level of sleep most necessary for cognitive restoration. In fact, some authorities (e.g., Horne, 1988) have referred to stages 1 and 2 as "optional sleep" that may not be as necessary to an individual as SWS or REM sleep. This assertion remains controversial, however, and the reader is referred to Horne (1991) and Carskadon and Roth (1991) for a full discussion of the issue.

Sleep Architecture

The two types and four stages of sleep do not occur randomly throughout the night, but have a typical pattern, or "architecture," to them. Though not entirely predictable, this regularity does allow researchers to observe when a particular pattern of sleep is in some way aberrant — an important ability when studying the sleep of shift workers.

For a healthy young day worker, the night usually starts with 90–100 minutes of SWS (following a 5- to 10-minute descent through the first two stages of sleep) [see Figure 5.2]. The first burst of REM sleep, which is usually less than 20 minutes long, then occurs. Thereafter, REM sleep bursts occur approximately every 90 minutes throughout the night (an ultradian rhythm — see Chapter 2), with each subsequent REM burst longer than the one before it. Simultaneously, the amount of SWS in non-REM sleep progressively declines during the night, until sleep is either stage 1, stage 2, or REM toward the end of the sleep period. The amount of REM sleep an individual gets appears to be governed by his or her circadian system (the biological clock), and REM sleep occurring early in the sleep episode has been viewed as an indication that the circadian system is not properly aligned for restful sleep and active wakefulness. SWS appears to be more homeostatically than rhythmically determined, being more of a function of the time since waking than of the phase of the circadian system at which it occurs (Anch et al., 1988).

The Sleep of a Shift Worker

Since the last thing most shift workers have time for is being wired for observation in a sleep laboratory, there are not many studies reporting the objectively measured sleep patterns of shift workers. In summarizing the results of the few studies that do exist, Akerstedt (1985) concluded that day sleep is one to four hours shorter than night sleep, with the reduction occurring primarily in stage 2 and REM sleep (SWS sleep remains relatively unaffected). REM sleep often occurs earlier in a day sleep episode than in night sleep, revealing patterns consistent with a circadian system that is not properly aligned for a restful period of sleep.

Although the abnormal sleep architecture of shift workers may indicate a lack of circadian adaptation, it is the shortened <u>duration</u> of sleep that is the most apparent problem to the individuals concerned. Nearly every survey of the problems associated with shift work (including our own interviews for this book) lists "getting enough sleep" as the number one problem.

Large-scale surveys of German and Japanese shift workers showed convincing evidence of a relationship between sleep length and bedtime (Kogi, 1985). Sleep lengths decrease as one moves from the early morning to mid-afternoon, and increase thereafter (see Figure 5.3). Some authors have suggested that much of this sleep truncation is self-inflicted, due to domestic commitments or a cavalier attitude by the shift worker and/or the family regarding the need for sleep (Tepas, Walsh, and Armstrong, 1981). Even in a soundproof laboratory with ad-lib sleep encouraged, however, sleep duration varies as a function of the time of day at which it is attempted. In a well-controlled study by Akerstedt and Gillberg (1981), morning bedtimes were associated with about 50% less sleep than late evening bedtimes, even after a night without sleep (see Figure 5.3). In such instances, the circadian system works to wake up the shift worker before sufficient sleep has been acquired. Therefore, although noise and family commitments are undoubtedly factors in the success or failure of day sleep, they are not the only ones — the status of the circadian system is one of the prime determinants of the amount of sleep obtained. This is a very important fact for the nurse shift worker to understand. All too often, sleep disruption is blamed on noises from the outside, when the real disruption is coming from the biological clock inside the shift worker's own head.

(One of the major goals of Chapter 8 is to help get the nurse shift worker's circadian system "set" right.)

Sleep and Aging

Sleep patterns change throughout the human life span. In general, the trend is a decline in the amount and quality of sleep as we age. There are two important points to consider with regard to sleep and aging:

1) Individuals in late adolescence are likely to need significantly more sleep than their adult counterparts, and should be encouraged (and allowed) to choose bedtimes and waketimes appropriately.
2) Late middle-aged and elderly individuals tend to experience more "fragile" sleep, with multiple awakenings and lighter sleep stages. This may intensify the sleep disruption consequent upon changing sleep-wake routines.

Additionally, other sleep pathologies are more likely to develop with age. The two most common are *sleep apnea* (a cessation of breathing during sleep) and *nocturnal myoclonus* (involuntary leg jerks during sleep), both of which can lead to an impaired ability to sleep without interruption. The transient sleep interruptions caused by these conditions usually are too brief to be remembered by the sleeper, but are frequent enough to be detrimental to waketime functioning (Neylan and Reynolds, 1991).

Naps

While regular afternoon napping is not part of the lives of most North Americans, it is an integral part of many other cultures around the world (Dinges and Broughton, 1989). A number of experiments have revealed a <u>universal</u> afternoon propensity to nap (Broughton, 1989; Campbell, 1984), which is present even if lunch is not taken and time cues are removed (Carskadon and Dement, 1992).

In a review of the napping literature, Dinges (1989) noted that most naps last between 40 and 90 minutes, with an overall mean of 73 minutes. The precise architecture of the nap (i.e., its patterning in terms of sleep stages and types) depends on the circadian timing of nap onset, and on the nap's duration and proximity to the major

47

sleep episode. For instance, REM sleep is likely to predominate when naps are taken in the rising phase of the circadian temperature cycle (i.e., in the morning hours for those with a day-oriented schedule).

Napping represents a double-edged sword with regard to sleep management. Although naps can be very useful in making up for previous sleep deficits and/or anticipated sleep loss (e.g., before a night shift), the major sleep episode may be less consolidated if napping has taken the edge off sleep need, and circadian rhythms may be disrupted by a multiphased sleep pattern. These findings make us cautious in our advice on napping for the nurse shift worker. We recommend that shift-working nurses use naps sparingly — perhaps napping before a run of night duty or as a topping-off process, but not as part of a regular daily routine. (More information on the relationship between napping and shift work is provided in Chapter 8.)

Summary

Sleep is an active, heterogenous process with different stages, types, and depths. The changing schedules of shift workers induce circadian dysfunction and disrupt both the architecture and amount of sleep. Moreover, sleep is heavily influenced by the circadian system and cannot simply be undertaken at will. Naps should be used cautiously, or they may disrupt the circadian system and interfere with the major sleep episode.

FIGURE 5.1
Typical Sleep EEG Polygraph Traces

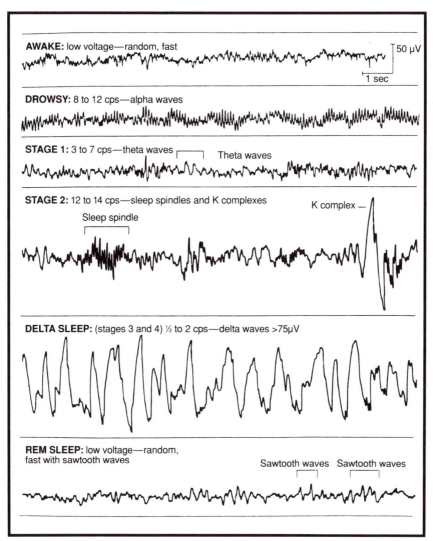

AWAKE: low voltage—random, fast

⌐ 50 µV

⌐ 1 sec

DROWSY: 8 to 12 cps—alpha waves

STAGE 1: 3 to 7 cps—theta waves | Theta waves

STAGE 2: 12 to 14 cps—sleep spindles and K complexes

Sleep spindle

K complex —

DELTA SLEEP: (stages 3 and 4) ½ to 2 cps—delta waves >75µV

REM SLEEP: low voltage—random,
fast with sawtooth waves

Sawtooth waves   Sawtooth waves

From Hauri, 1982.

FIGURE 5.2
Typical Sleep Histogram

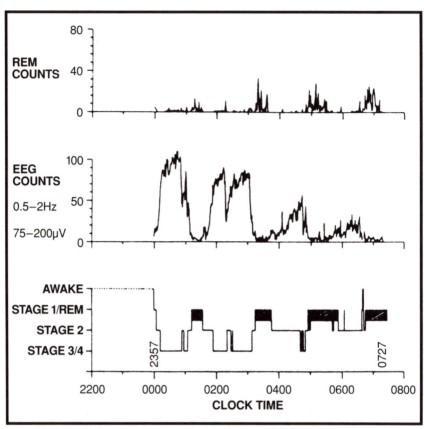

This typical sleep histogram represents a healthy young male subject studied in Dr. Monk's laboratory. The upper panel shows the occurrence of REM activity; the middle panel shows the pattern of delta activity; and the bottom panel shows the actual patterning of sleep through the night.

FIGURE 5.3
Relationship Between Bedtime and Sleep Length

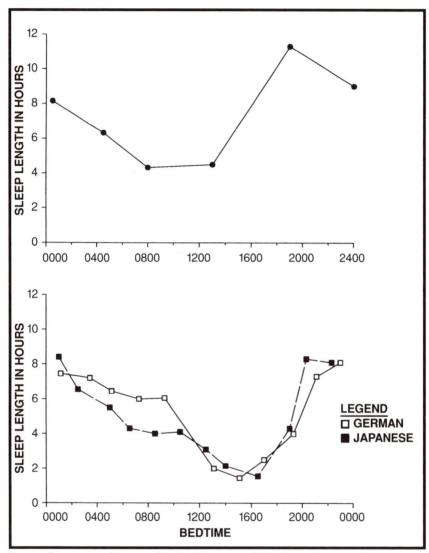

Top graph represents the mean of six healthy young adult subjects; lower graph represents data from 2,332 German and 3,240 Japanese shift workers. In all cases, morning bedtimes followed a night without sleep. From Akerstedt and Gillberg, 1981 (top); and Kogi, 1985 (bottom).

— Chapter 6 —

Performance at Night

Introduction

Despite a natural reluctance on the part of some employers and labor unions to suffer the inconvenience of participating in shift work research, the performance of night shift workers has received a fair amount of attention from the chronobiological and chronopsychological scientific communities. Nurses have been the subject of quite a few studies because they provide an excellent opportunity to evaluate whether there are measurable shift performance differences among a largely female working population. In contrast to many other fields, the health care industry, and particularly the nursing profession, provides researchers with night shift subjects who work rapid, weekly, or slow rotation patterns, as well as 8- and 12-hour permanent shift schedules, within a single institution.

Testifying on shift work before a Congressional subcommittee in the early 1980s, an American Nurses Association spokesperson stressed the need for research into the relationship between the physiological and psychological effects of shift rotation on nurses and the quality of nursing care delivered to hospital patients (Panel investigates, 1983). Perhaps because of the large number of uncontrolled variables that make shift work research difficult, or even personal aversions to night work, only a few nurse researchers responded to this call, as evidenced by the paucity of published nursing research reports on the topic.

The current focus on continuous quality improvement programs within the health care community does not include methods to differentiate the quality of nursing care that patients receive on day, evening, and night shifts. Even data on such easily documented incidents as the number of medication errors on day, evening, and night shifts were not available from the nursing departments we polled in our earlier studies (Alward, 1986; Alward and Monk, 1990). Although the annual performance evaluations of permanent night and evening shift nurses can be used as measures of performance on those shifts, the evaluations of rotating night shift nurses cannot similarly be used since they also measure performance on other shifts.

Direct observational measurement of nurses' night work performance is the ideal method of study, but the practical problems involved are immense for a large sample of nurses. (So many observers are needed and nurses' work is so varied that the task becomes unmanageable.) Most of the few published studies on night work that we discuss in this chapter have measured the performance of night shift nurses through indirect means, such as supervisors' ratings or self-appraisals. Although some research has measured nurses' performance on artificial tasks (Hawkins and Armstrong-Esther, 1978), such studies are often perceived by nurses as artificial and/or irrelevent, and therefore lack validity. Even if a standard test could be developed for the wide variety of professional nurses, the problems of practice effects (the effects of repeated practice on test results), test anxiety, and time involved in testing remain significant barriers.

Until these research difficulties can be resolved, there are some general findings regarding shift worker performance that can be applied to night shift nursing, with the following precautions. It should be remembered that these studies are mainly concerned with male shift workers in industrialized settings, whose biological, psychosocial, and work characteristics might be rather different than those of the predominantly female nursing population. Also, although there is a recent trend toward more activity at night, night shift work is qualitatively different than day shift work for many nurses.

The conceptual model represented in Figure 6.1 (like the later model developed by DeVries-Griever and Meijman, 1987) illustrates that the on-shift performance of the shift worker is the product of many different factors — some interacting directly, others operating through changes in the shift adjustment process. This model reinforces the point that measuring nurses' on-shift performance is a complex task.

Circadian Performance Rhythms

The study of diurnal variation in human performance has an illustrious history, predating the coinage of the term "circadian" by half a century (Lavie, 1980). By the late-1960s, the dominant theory of diurnal variation was of a single performance rhythm, usually parallel to the temperature rhythm (Colquhoun, 1971) — except in memory tasks such as digit span (the number of random digits that can be recalled from memory), the rhythms of which were explained in terms of superoptimal arousal (Blake, 1967) [see below]. For some tasks (such as searching through lists), the parallelism with temperature rhythm is quite striking, with both showing a rise over the waking day (see Figure 6.2). The single performance rhythm theory persisted until the mid-1970s, when Folkard (1975) studied the time-of-day effect in two complex cognitive tasks — solving logical syllogisms and the Baddeley (1968) logical reasoning test. These tasks represented a departure from previous studies (Blake, 1967) in that, unlike simple reaction and card-sorting tasks, they involved the subjects in fairly complex thought processes and could not simply be worked through automatically in a mindless, routine manner. Folkard's results reveal time-of-day curves with a midday peak, showing thought processes to be fastest around noon (see Figure 6.3), unlike either the digit span or simple repetitive task time-of-day results. This discovery heralded a new approach to the study of circadian performance rhythms, with more emphasis on the differences between circadian performance rhythms than on their similarities, and on the mechanisms by which circadian performance rhythms might occur.

Later circadian performance rhythms research focused on memory tasks (Folkard and Monk, 1985). It was clear even from the early studies that the time-of-day function for memory tasks was very different from that for other tasks. Research by Baddeley et al. (1970) and Hockey, Davies, and Gray (1972) confirmed that for relatively "pure" tasks involving immediate memory (e.g., memory tested within a few minutes of a presentation), performance was better in the morning than in either the afternoon or evening. This result was

explained in terms of the Arousal Model, by postulating that immediate memory was interfered with by the higher levels of arousal
believed to occur in the evening (Hockey and Colquhoun, 1972).
However, this does not work for all types of memory. Although
high arousal is bad for short-term memory, it is good for long-term
memory. For example, we tend to remember scary situations rather
well. Thus, our naturally higher arousal in the afternoon or evening
might be better for committing material to long-term memory than
our lower arousal in the morning. This finding was first confirmed
in a study of schoolchildren's memories of a story presented at either
9:00 a.m. (low arousal) or 3:30 p.m. (high arousal). Immediate memory was better for material heard at 9:00 a.m., and delayed (one
week) memory was better for material heard at 3:30 p.m. (Folkard
et al., 1977). Further confirmation was provided through a study of
night shift nurses' memories of a training film presented at either
8:30 p.m. or 4:00 a.m. Although night shift nurses whose rhythms
were not adjusted to night work showed better immediate retention
of the material at 4:00 a.m. than at 8:30 p.m., their delayed retention
(tested one month later) was the reverse, with the 8:30 p.m. presentation being superior (Monk and Folkard, 1978).

For tasks such as monitoring and inspection that do not involve
memory, performance is largely predictable from the body temperature rhythm, with poor performance occurring at or near the trough
in body temperature, which occurs for day workers in the early
hours of the morning (Colquhoun, 1971). For the night-working
nurse, this means that there is likely to be a 4:00–6:00 a.m. slump in
monitoring performance. This finding is confirmed in the six studies
that have been able to obtain relatively continuous, 24-hour data
from actual work performance in various occupations. These studies, which show a remarkable similarity in time-of-day function (see
Figure 6.4), can be divided into three that measure the speed
(Browne, 1949; Wojtczak-Jaroszowa and Pawlowksa-Skyba, 1967) or
accuracy (Bjerner and Swensson, 1953) with which the primary task
is performed, and three that measure the consequences of lapses in
attention or vigilance (Folkard and Monk, 1979; Hildebrandt, Rohmert, and Rutenfranz, 1974; Prokop and Prokop, 1955). All six studies show performance of these tasks to be worse during the night
hours, although in three of the studies there is also evidence of a
pronounced post-lunch dip that almost equals the nighttime dip.
(Many of us are aware of this early afternoon slump in our alertness.) Additionally, a study of truck drivers confirms the risk of acci-

dents between midnight and 2:00 a.m. to be more than double the normal risk (Hamelin, 1987).

In general, we see that different tasks exhibit "best" and "worst" times of day. Those that do not involve short-term memory are usually predictable in their circadian rhythm from the rhythm in body temperature, which exhibits a trough around 4:00 a.m. and a peak around 8:00 p.m. in day workers and unadjusted shift workers. Additionally, some tasks might exhibit a post-lunch dip in the early afternoon.

Night Shift Performance

The job performance of nurses in relation to their hours of work and type of shift system has been investigated by several researchers, and is summarized in this section. The results of these studies consistently confirm that rotating shift nurses generally do not perform as well as permanent night shift nurses, although none of the studies compared strictly-defined rapidly rotating shift nurses to permanent shift nurses. In reviewing the results of these studies, it is important to remember that most nursing organizations rarely adhere to rigid shift rotation patterns; therefore, samples of rotating shift nurses often represent a mixture of unspecified rotation speeds and schedules.

In the large NIOSH study of the health consequences of shift work, Tasto and Colligan (1978) studied 1,049 registered nurses and licensed practical nurses, divided into four shift groups: permanent day, permanent evening, permanent night, and all rotating shifts. The rotating shift nurses consistently fared the worst in aspects of physical and psychological health, job satisfaction, and self-rated performance, followed closely by fixed night shift nurses. No information was provided about the frequency of rotation, or whether both rapid and slow rotation systems were used.

The attendance records of a slightly larger sample of nurses analyzed in the same study showed that the group of rotating shift nurses tended to take more sick leave than the three groups of permanent shift nurses, while the permanent night shift nurses tended to take more sick leave than either the permanent day or evening groups (Tasto and Colligan, 1978). Rotating shift nurses also tended to give more serious reasons for sick leave, and had significantly more clinic visits and accidents during the six months of study than did the fixed shift nurses. In both instances, there was a lot of variability in the data and the conclusions were not very reliable.

Jamal and Jamal (1982) studied the job performance of 440 Canadian nurses, comparing a group of fixed shift nurses with a group of rotating shift nurses. Because of the small samples of permanent night shift ($n = 14$) and evening shift ($n = 31$) nurses, these subjects were combined with the permanent day shift nurses to form one group of permanent shift nurses ($n = 245$). The rotating shift nurses were also combined into one group. When the supervisors' ratings of job performance, job motivation, and patient care factors were statistically analyzed, significantly better performance in the fixed shift group was found for all three performance factors.

The supervisory rating scale developed by Jamal and Jamal (1982) was selected as a measure of nurses' performance when Dr. Alward (1986) compared 38 permanent night shift nurses with 38 rotating night shift nurses. The nurses were compared on a series of measures theoretically linked with night work performance, including self-reported adaptation to night work, fatigue, general activation (how wide awake they were), stress, absence behavior, sleepiness, and quantity of sleep obtained. Permanent night shift nurses demonstrated significantly higher supervisors' ratings, greater adaptation to night work, and less fatigue. The findings suggested that, at least in this sample, permanent night shift nurses may perform better than rotating night shift nurses who work at least three consecutive night shifts. All nurses in this study were female RNs under 46 years old who worked eight-hour shifts at the same hospital. To control for differences in work characteristics, critical care nurses were not included in the sample.

In a third North American study, Coffey, Skipper, and Jung (1988) compared four groups of RNs' ($N = 463$) self-reported ratings on Schwirian's (1978) Six-Dimension Scale of Nursing Performance. Overall job performance was highest for the day shift group and lowest for the rotating shift group. The correlation between shift work and overall performance was statistically significant, although not strong. When comparing the four nursing groups' self-ratings on the five subscales of Schwirian's model, only the areas of professional development and leadership were associated with the types of shift systems worked. For both of these areas, permanent day and night shift workers rated themselves higher than did rotating or evening shift nurses.

In a British study that supported using permanent night shift nurses rather than rotating night shift nurses, the alertness levels of two groups of student nurses were compared by measuring performance at 10:30 p.m. and 3:30 a.m. on a simple reaction time test (responding quickly to a signal) [Wilkinson and Allison, 1989]. The rotating shift group worked a week of night duty, followed by six days off duty and from 3–15 weeks of day duty, before rotating to another week of night shifts. This group was compared to student nurses working three months of continuous night shifts, which involved cycles of three or four nights on duty, followed by three or four days off duty. The rotating shift group exhibited more drowsiness (i.e., responded more slowly) at the 3:30 a.m. testing on the seventh night than on the first night of work. The fixed night shift group did not show increased drowsiness on their last night of the three-month work period, although reaction times slowed at the midpoint of the three-month assignment. The researchers concluded that permanent night shifts are generally more conducive to optimum performance than weekly rotation, despite considerable individual differences in alertness among members of both groups. This study did not address the validity of using simple reaction time tests to approximate alertness and drowsiness during actual nursing performance.

A group of Boston scientists recently reported the results of their investigation of the relationship of work schedules to nurses' sleep schedules, sleepiness levels, and accident rates at work and while driving home (Gold et al., 1992). The subjects of this study were 593 female RNs and 42 female LPNs. Nurses who rotated between day and evening shifts reported getting more hours of sleep than either the permanent or rotating night shift nurses. Compared to the day/evening shift nurses, the rotating night shift group had twice the amount of reported errors and accidents at work or while driving home. The rotating night shift nurses also had 2.5 times more reported near-miss accidents. Both permanent night and rotating night shift nurses reported a significantly poorer quality of sleep, more use of medications to sleep, and more frequent nodding off while driving to or from work than did the day/evening shift group. Nodding off on the night shift occurred at least once a week for 32.4% of the permanent night shift nurses and for 35.3% of the rotating night shift nurses. Only 2.8% of the day/evening nurses nodded off while on duty. For most categories of accidents and errors investigated, rotating shift night nurses fared somewhat worse than permanent night shift nurses. All data were self-reported by the nurses and could not be validated.

Night Shift Paralysis

Folkard, Condon, and Herbert (1984) have described a syndrome they call *night shift paralysis*. In their survey of 434 British night shift nurses, 12% of the nurses reported experiencing, at least once or twice in their work lives, a temporary paralysis that totally incapacitated them for an average of four minutes. This night shift paralysis typically occurred around 4:00 a.m. while the nurses sat at a desk, and the likelihood of paralysis tended to increase over consecutive night shifts of work. Most of the nurses reporting this syndrome were under 30 years old.

In a similar study of 435 air traffic controllers from 17 countries, 6% reported one or more episodes of night shift paralysis in their work lives, lasting an average of two minutes. Although victims of this syndrome were conscious of their surroundings, they were not able to move. The researchers identified the following contributing factors:

- time of night,
- number of consecutive shifts worked,
- rigid sleeping habits, and
- working both a morning and night shift on the same day.

Twelve of the total 75 incidents reported by the air traffic controllers occurred during the day shift (Folkard and Condon, 1987).

The incidence of night shift paralysis is thought to be an indication of high levels of sleepiness. Because of the obvious threat to nursing performance and patient safety, we encourage nurse researchers to investigate both the incidence and prevention of the consequences of sleep deprivation.

Patient Care at Night

While nurses have been the primary subject of a limited number of shift work studies, clinical nursing practice and patient needs during the night have received very little attention from nurse researchers. We found no studies that asked patients how satisfied they were with nursing care at night.

In many U.S. hospitals, nursing activity at night has changed significantly since the early 1980s as patient acuity and severity-of-illness indices have increased. Many medical-surgical units now resemble the critical care units of 20 years ago. Night shift nurses and their managers increasingly report less free time; the 2:00–4:00 a.m. "quiet time" for updating charts no longer exists. Night shift nursing demands more critical thinking and decision-making skills than ever before, and the work of hospital night shift nurses in the United States can no longer be thought of as being involved primarily with vigilance tasks.

The one constant in night shift nursing seems to be that patients still complain of noise on nursing units at night, and of being awakened unnecessarily. An English nurse indicted the nursing profession for undervaluing the benefits of patients' sleep and not treating sleep importantly enough in daily patient care planning (Kemp, 1984). We only hope that the growing emphasis on continuous quality improvement has led to changes in this situation, and we look forward to more sleep research related to patient care.

Summary

Performance at night is not simply a problem of having to perform at the "down phase" of the circadian cycle. Night shift nurses also must take into account the nature of the task to be performed and the decreases in performance that result from chronic jet-lag-type symptoms, partial sleep loss, and decrements in mood and well-being. The "end result" performance, therefore, will be determined by many factors, some relating directly and others relating indirectly through changes in mood and motivation.

FIGURE 6.1
A Conceptual Model of the Factors Affecting On-Shift Performance

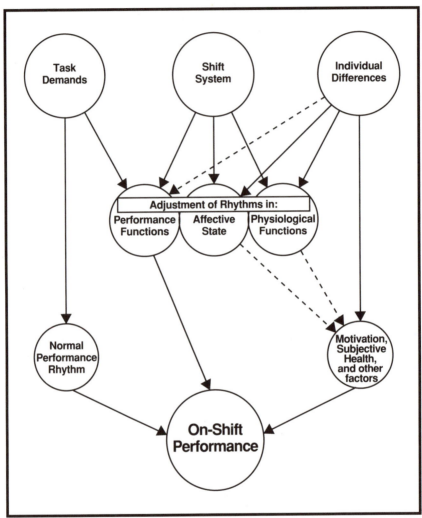

Solid lines represent known influences affecting on-shift performance; dashed lines represent probable influences. From Folkard and Monk, 1979.

FIGURE 6.2
Time-of-Day Effects in Search Tasks

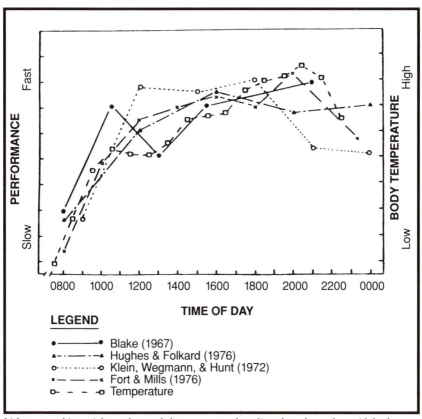

LEGEND

- •———• Blake (1967)
- ▲–·—·–▲ Hughes & Folkard (1976)
- ○·········○ Klein, Wegmann, & Hunt (1972)
- ×— — —× Fort & Mills (1976)
- □– – – –□ Temperature

24-hour trend in serial search speed, from a range of studies plotted together with body temperature. From Monk, 1979.

FIGURE 6.3
Time-of-Day Function for Performance in Logical Syllogism and Grammatical Transformation Tasks

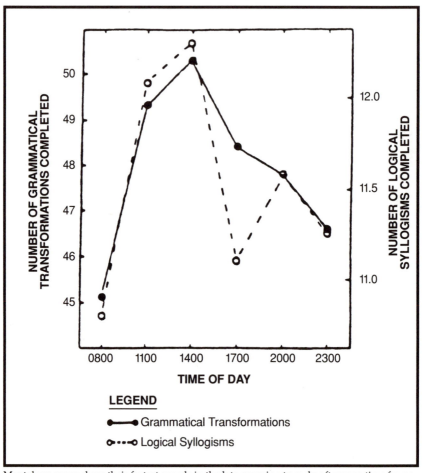

Mental processes show their fastest speeds in the late-morning to early-afternoon time frame. From Folkard, 1975.

FIGURE 6.4
Variations in "Real Work" Performance Measures Over a 24-Hour Day

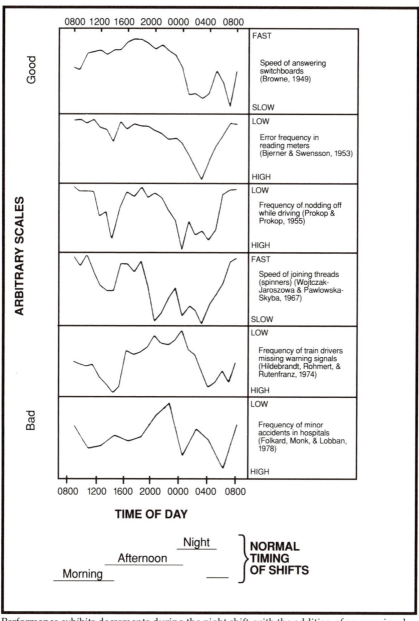

Performance exhibits decrements during the night shift, with the addition of an occasional mid-afternoon slump. From Folkard and Monk, 1979.

Chapter 7

Shift Work Assessment

Introduction

Assessment is the first step in the clinical problem-solving process so familiar to nurses. Similarly, before nurse shift workers can learn to cope with their work schedules, they must become familiar with shift work assessment techniques. As far as we know, health care institutions generally do not provide any preemployment screening or health surveillance for shift maladaptation syndrome, although some nurse employers (very few, unfortunately) do sponsor in-service education on shift work adaptation. For the vast majority of night and rotating shift nurses, assessing tolerance to shift work and planning adaptation strategies are personal responsibilities. Most of the nurses we interviewed for this book received no assistance in this process, and were eager to share their problems and success stories.

When an individual follows a regular daily schedule, there are consistent trough and peak times for all circadian rhythms, which run in synchrony with each other. Although the self-sustaining circadian system is resistant to change, disruptions in activity patterns or social routines can cause uncoupling of the individual rhythms. *External desynchronization* occurs when a conflict arises between an individual's internal circadian rhythms and external zeitgebers such as social activities or light-dark cycles. The phenomenon of rhythms peaking at abnormal times in relation to each other is called *internal dissociation*. The stress caused by external desynchronization and internal dissociation can have negative effects on the nurse shift worker's performance and general well-being. Therefore, some background information on the shift work adaptation process can help nurse shift workers set goals to enable their circadian systems to function as well as possible.

Sleep, body temperature, and neuroendocrine rhythms are the most important of the physiological rhythms that must adjust to the inverted work schedule of the night shift nurse. The rate at which individual circadian rhythms adjust to an altered schedule is not consistent. For example, as mentioned in Chapter 2, the body temperature rhythm usually takes much longer to completely adjust to a change in schedule than does the sleep-wake cycle.

The daily rhythmic fluctuations in psychological variables — such as mood, vigor, arousal, alertness, activation, time estimation, and memory — also have been found to require different amounts of time to adapt to an acute time shift in the sleep-activity cycle. Because performance measures cannot be studied during the hours of sleep, trends in performance are referred to as *diurnal variations* or *time-of-day effects* rather than as circadian rhythms. As we discussed in Chapter 6, changes in performance levels during the workday are assumed to reflect underlying circadian rhythms. Folkard and Monk (1979) point out that it is no easy task to assess the relationship between shift work and performance. One must take into account variations in work demands, sleep schedules, health and motivation levels, social activities, and family and economic circumstances, as well as individual differences in normal circadian rhythm parameters and adaptability to changes in work routines.

In this chapter, we will discuss some of the issues that affect the shift work adaptation process, and will suggest how nurses can initiate a self-assessment of suitability for shift work. We will offer suggestions to assist the nurse shift worker in setting and meeting circadian system goals through choosing a shift system, assessing sleep patterns, making any necessary social adjustments, and managing time. We will conclude this chapter with methods to assess shift work strengths and weaknesses by considering circadian type, age, experience, and social responsibilities. The shift work adaptation program presented in Chapter 8 describes further interventions to facilitate shift work adaptation, which should be based on the assessment techniques presented in this chapter.

Shift Work Adaptation Factors

In Chapter 4, we outlined some of the health problems that impede adaptation to night and rotating shift work. Certain individual characteristics and social factors are also known to influence adaptation to and tolerance of shift work. Scott and LaDou (1990) include the following relative contraindications for shift work:

- being over 40 years old,
- extreme "morningness,"
- sleep rigidity,
- family instability,
- excessive family responsibilities, and/or
- a lengthy work commute.

Many of these social factors and individual characteristics are related to sleep deficits in shift workers. As with existing health disorders, the shift worker's level of commitment and success in adopting and maintaining a compatible routine help negate the effects of the contraindications. The higher the shift worker's motivation to adapt, the greater the likelihood that ways will be found to adjust to the work schedule.

While age and individual factors such as circadian type, sleep needs, and personality cannot be altered, other variables such as health status, work experience, and behavior patterns are amenable to change (usually, however, only with considerable effort). It is important, therefore, that employers and employees know where to focus their adaptation efforts. For instance, the work schedule itself can be manipulated to facilitate either adaptation or nonadaptation. (Nonadaptation might very well be the goal of the rotating shift nurse who works three 12-hour night shifts during a one-week period, and then cycles to a month of 12-hour day shifts.) Additionally, the nurse's sleep, eating, exercise, and social schedules can be adjusted to facilitate circadian rhythm adaptation.

An important assessment question that must be answered by any nurse considering shift work is: "How much am I willing to adjust my sleep patterns, my dietary habits, my physical activity routine, and my social life in order to adapt to shift work?" If the answer is "not much," we would advise the nurse either to seek day or evening shift work, or to stick with rapid shift rotations, which do not allow time for the circadian system to change its internal phase (although, for many nurses, rapid rotation through the night shift can entail significant performance deficits and fatigue).

Setting Circadian System Goals

The primary goal of both permanent night shift nurses and those rotating shift nurses whose schedules include night work is to adapt to the acute time shifts in their sleep-activity cycles as quickly as possible. Adaptation techniques may vary considerably for the nurses on these two different shift systems. For permanent night shift nurses and those nurses who work slowly rotating shifts, the goal is to invert their circadian rhythms, resynchronize them to an inverted night-work/day-sleep schedule, and maintain that condition for as long as necessary. For the rapidly rotating night shift nurse who works two nights before reverting to a day or evening schedule, the goal is to remain synchronized to a diurnal schedule, tolerating the temporarily disrupted sleep-activity cycle as well as possible.

Choosing a Shift System

The nursing divisions of most U.S. hospitals have a variety of shift systems in place throughout their departments and units. Certain work schedules may be more suitable than others for individual nurses due to physiological, psychological, performance, and/or social reasons. In order to determine the shift that is best suited to their needs, shift-working nurses should answer the following assessment questions:

- Which types of shift systems are used on this unit?
- What hours will I be expected to work?
- Can I review sample work schedules for typical shift rotation patterns on this unit?
- Do contractual agreements govern shift work and rotation policies on this unit? If so, can I review sample agreements?
- What other types of shift systems are used throughout the institution?
- What type of food service is available during the night shift?

- When are in-service education classes offered to evening and night shift personnel?
- Are staff meetings held on the evening and night shifts?
- What is the pay differential for working evening and night shifts?

A nurse accepting rotating shift work should query the interviewer and examine a number of sample work schedules in order to answer the following questions:

- Will I be expected to rotate to all three shifts, or to only two shifts? (Days-to-evenings or days-to-nights are common rotation patterns in most nursing organizations.)
- If nurses on this unit rotate to all three shifts, is the order of rotation the recommended clockwise direction of days-to-evenings-to-nights? (Phase delays are better tolerated by most shift-working nurses than phase advances, which are represented by counterclockwise shift rotations of days-to-nights-to-evenings.)
- Does shift rotation on this unit follow a regular pattern?
- Is shift rotation rapid, slow, or both?
- If shift rotation is slow, does the schedule allow <u>at least</u> two weeks between shift changes? (At best, it takes two to three weeks for the human circadian system to adapt to night work. Experts agree that a one-week shift rotation schedule is the most difficult for circadian system adaptation [U.S. Congress, 1991].)

Both permanent and rotating shift nurses need to know if they will have a choice of shift lengths, and if self-scheduling is practiced. Successfully inverting circadian rhythms will be improbable for nurses who work 12-hour night shifts because they are less likely to maintain a daytime sleep schedule on nonworking days. On the other hand, some nurses told us that they were less tired when working 12-hour night shifts because they could sleep more night-time hours on this compressed work schedule. Self-scheduling is preferred by most nurses because it allows them more control over days off work and a greater opportunity to make their professional and personal schedules compatible.

Answering these shift assessment questions will help both experienced and inexperienced staff nurses determine whether the shift systems used by an employing health care facility are compatible with their personal physiological, psychological, performance, social, and economic needs. If a nurse accepts a shift work position, the answers to the assessment questions also will help determine whether circadian system goals should be centered around inverting and then maintaining a resynchronized system, or around remaining on a diurnal schedule while trying to get enough sleep to function well during night shifts. Additionally, it is important for nurse managers to be aware of the shift work policies of the units they supervise, and to know whether these policies can be changed if they do not promote the well-being of individual nurse shift workers.

Assessing Sleep Patterns

All shift-working nurses should assess their individual sleep characteristics and requirements in order to form goals and plans that will accelerate shift work adaptation. The nurses we interviewed for this book had not undertaken formal sleep assessments; however, through trial and error, some of the permanent night shift nurses had arrived at strategies to improve the quality and quantity of their sleep. By experimenting with progressively later bedtimes after night shifts, several nurses came to the conclusion that they slept longer and better when they postponed sleep onset until the afternoon (this is not usually the case, however — see Chapter 8). Other nurses found it necessary to take a two- to four-hour evening nap before each night shift, both to ward off on-shift sleepiness and to obtain enough sleep.

In addition to determining when they prefer to sleep, shift-working nurses also must determine how much sleep they need. Sleep requirements vary greatly: some individuals function well with five hours of sleep, while others suffer if they get much less than 10–11 hours of sleep. Nurses who require 9–11 hours of sleep should consider working evening shifts; even those who work day shifts may find their sleep needs unmet unless they go to bed around 8:00 p.m. Few night shift nurses report sleeping over 7.5 hours per day. Nurses who complain of fatigue and poor quality of sleep may need more sleep than the average adult, and will rarely find these symptoms improved after starting shift work.

As pointed out in Chapter 5, night shift workers rarely have enough free time to participate in the objective measurement of their sleep patterns in a laboratory setting. Regardless, individual shift workers still can effectively assess their own sleep patterns by recording when they go to sleep and awaken on days both on and off duty. Tepas and Carvalhais (1990) report a high correlation between subjective reports of sleep length and polysomnographic recordings of sleep. Keeping a sleep log and self-evaluating sleep quality may seem to be bothersome at first, but will benefit the nurse who is concerned with sleep hygiene in the long run. Figure 7.1 presents a sample sleep diary, and a "Sleep Quality Questionnaire" is outlined in Figure 7.2. The tools presented in these two figures will help both permanent and rotating shift nurses assess the quality and quantity of their sleep in relationship to time of sleep onset and sleep interruptions, as well as to sleepiness and fatigue while on duty. For nurses who have firmly established routines for days both on and off duty, there may be no need to keep a sleep diary if assessment questions about sleep onset and waketimes can be easily answered.

Making Social Adjustments

The necessity of making social adjustments is often cited by nurses as one of the most unacceptable aspects of shift work. Many nurses choose permanent night shifts in order to spend more time with their children and to avoid the costs of day care. Making time for spouses, children, and friends may be more valuable to a nurse shift worker than sleep, even when sleep deprivation and chronic fatigue result from a shift work schedule. Arlene is an example of a nurse who chose to work permanent night shifts so that she could provide child care for her two sons. For eight years she existed by sleeping from 8:00–10:00 p.m. before her night shift, and napping when she could during her lunch break at night and during the day at home. As the numbers of dual-career and single parent families increase, and as sleep deprivation and social problems related to shift work multiply, there will be a greater need for self-assessments and adjustments within the social units of shift-working nurses.

When a choice of shift system is possible, nurses should consider social priorities and personal goals when making a selection. Permanent evening shifts diminish the time available for interaction with school-age children, dinners with family and friends, and participation in professional and community organizations. Permanent night shifts allow more time for social interactions, but often at the expense of the physiological circadian rhythm desynchrony that results from an inconsistent pattern of activity and sleep. If a night shift nurse's sexual partner works days, special effort may be required to avoid sexual dissatisfaction in the relationship. As pointed out in Chapter 3, rotating shift schedules also interfere with social and professional activities. The inconsistency of many nursing shift rotations makes simple survival the most common goal.

Few studies have been done on the impact of shift work on social and family adjustment among shift workers. Comparisons need to be made between shift workers' and day workers' rates of divorce, marital counseling, and psychotherapy, as well as of the delinquency, truancy, and academic problems of their children (Colligan and Rosa, 1990). We do know that preexisting patterns of communication, domestic task definition and sharing, and time management are important factors in the nurse shift worker's social adjustment, and in providing the sort of environment in which sleep and biological clock and adjustment goals can also be met. Family and friends need to know what is happening and what the problem areas are for the shift worker. Sleep, family interaction, and domestic chores all must have time specifically reserved for them. Everyone in the household must know their domestic responsibilities and when they are to be performed. Setting circadian system goals for a satisfactory adaptation to shift work requires an awareness and assessment of these factors as they relate to the nurse's social priorities and the attitudes and support of family and friends.

Nurses making career or shift work choices will want to consider the advantages and disadvantages of each available shift system in light of social, professional, domestic, and economic priorities. The following questions can assist nurses in a social and professional self-assessment of their shift work adaptability:

- When do you most want to be off duty?
- If a fixed day shift position is not available as your first choice, would fixed afternoon or night shifts be preferable to shift rotation (which may be very irregular)?
- Are 12-hour shifts an option for you? What are the advantages and disadvantages of a compressed work week?
- Are you willing to give up a secondary (moonlighting) position if that job adds stress to your shift work adaptation process?

- Will this shift work position be advantageous or detrimental to your long-term career goals?
- Will this position provide opportunities for social and professional networking?
- Are your family, friends, and colleagues committed to the changes that will be required in their lives and to the social support you will need in order to adapt to your shift work schedule and to stay socially and professionally connected?
- Will your sexual partner be cooperative and supportive in adjusting to changes in your social and sleeping schedules?
- Do you have hobbies or interests (such as writing, reading, gardening, or sewing) that will be compatible with your shift work schedule?

Time Management Strategies

Time management is a universal problem for nurses, whatever their positions or working hours. There never seems to be enough time for everything we want to do in our personal and professional lives, and so we learn to set goals and priorities in order to control the time we have and gain the results most important to us. Similar to controlling sleep patterns in order to gain the most vitality, nurses must first assess how their time is spent before it can be controlled. Once again, we recommend maintaining a time log (similar to the sleep diary outlined in Figure 7.1) to clearly illustrate how much time is spent on activities considered unimportant or unproductive, so that such activities eventually can be minimized or eliminated. In our interviews with night shift nurses, it was very apparent that the nurses who were most satisfied with shift work were those who effectively managed their time.

In an article for nurse managers on ways to assess and change time-wasting behaviors, Eliopoulos (1984) begins a list of general rules with, "Know your body clock." Adding to her suggestions, we offer the following general guidelines for effective time management (the Circadian Type Questionnaire presented in Figure 7.3 will help with this assessment):

- Know when your energy levels are highest and lowest.
- Know at what time of day you best retain information.

- Know when your post-lunch energy dip occurs.
- Know when your body temperatures are highest and lowest.
- Know when you prefer to go to sleep and awaken.
- Know when you most enjoy eating meals.
- Control your daily schedule and limit interruptions. Learn to say no. Allow time in your schedule for those activities most important to you, including personal relaxation and professional enhancement activities (essential for the night shift nurse who must follow a rather rigid schedule in order to maintain optimal functioning and general well-being).
- Set realistic goals for yourself and do not accept more responsibility than you can manage. Remember that working at night may substantially reduce productivity, especially during shift adaptation periods.
- Do not procrastinate, as it only compounds the work to which you must eventually respond.

Assessing Your Circadian Type

While managing time, adjusting social habits, and modifying sleep patterns are tangible goals nurse shift workers can achieve in the quest for shift work adaptation, some other individual differences are less amenable to change, such as *circadian type,* or *chronotype.* As early as 1939, Kleitman (1963) identified morning and evening chronotypes through differences in peak body temperatures and sensory/perceptual performance times. Through questionnaires and physiological and psychological measures, we have learned that morning types (larks) have earlier peaking daily rhythms (e.g., body temperature) than evening types (owls); more importantly, morning types have a significantly greater problem coping with night shift work and changes in sleeping times. Not only do larks find it harder than owls to remain alert at night, but sleep during the day is more difficult for larks and the time cues of a day-oriented society are more pressing (Monk and Folkard, 1992).

Before accepting a shift work assignment, nurses should assess their individual circadian type. The Circadian Type Questionnaire (CTQ) can help with the assessment and planning phases in a shift work adaptation progrm (see Figure 7.3), although it is not meant to be used as a management tool. It is important to remember that the CTQ measures probabilities rather than absolutes, and that many other factors must be considered in evaluating tolerance for and adjustment to nursing shift work (Alward, 1988). We should also point out that only a small percentage of people fall into extreme circadian type categories — most of us fall near the middle of the morningness-eveningness continuum.

In the late-1970s, Drs. Simon Folkard and Mary Lobban worked with Dr. Monk to develop the CTQ as a measure of shift work suitability. Using a sample of 48 night shift nurses, they identified rigidity/flexibility of sleep habits (Rs), ability/inability to overcome drowsiness (V), and morningness/eveningness (M) as the three main factors distinguishing nurses whose circadian rhythms had adjusted to night work from those whose circadian rhythms had not adjusted (Folkard, Monk, and Lobban, 1979). In general, lower Rs scores (indicating more flexible sleeping habits) and higher V scores (indicating more vigor) were associated with better physiological circadian rhythm adjustment. Regularity of sleep habits (i.e., adhering to the same bedtime on workdays, weekends, and vacations) was a particularly strong indicator of those nurses likely to have shift work coping problems. The nurses categorized as "rigid sleepers" tended to report more disturbing noises while trying to sleep than those nurses who were more flexible in their sleeping habits, even though the sleeping accommodations and noise levels for the two groups were equivalent.

Age and Experience

Age plays a major role in differentiating those who can from those who cannot adjust to shift work. In general, as one gets older, shift work problems become more acute. The reason for this is that the biological clock changes with age, especially after reaching 40, when morning sleep becomes more difficult and the biological clock becomes harder to reset and less robust in its troughs and peaks. Sleep itself becomes more fragile — more easily disrupted, with less of the deepest stages of sleep (stages 3 and 4) — even for day workers (see Chapter 5). Health problems also can start to appear after age 40, adding extra stress to an already difficult situation. These facts may explain why a relatively small percentage of nurses remain on shift work until normal retirement age.

Less well-known is evidence that, independent of age, the subjective quality of sleep decreases as years of shift work experience increase. In a study of 700 French oil refinery employees, this finding was most striking in the group of workers who were between 51 and 65 years old (Foret et al., 1981). In this group, 65% of those with less than four years of shift work experience rated their sleep quality good, while 6% rated it poor. For those who had 27–41 years of shift work experience, 39% rated their sleep quality good, while 13% rated it poor. During vacations, sleep quality was related only to age, regardless of the years of shift work experience. We are not aware of a similar study using nurse subjects, but the results of this French study provide added information to factor into a nurse's shift work self-assessment.

Because adaptability to shift work may change with age and experience, nurses should consider the assessment of tolerance to shift work as an ongoing process and not just a one-time event. For example, Janice has worked as a night shift nursing supervisor for many years, but after she turned 51, her work hours and commute became intolerable. Although her home is quieter now than when her three children were growing up, sleep has become more difficult, of shorter duration, and of poorer quality. Janice recently had an accident driving home from work, and has had to pull over to the side of the road because of acute sleepiness on several occasions. She has developed a duodenal ulcer that has not responded to medication, and is scheduled for a gastric resection. Clearly, Janice needs to assess her career options and determine whether she can continue to cope with the stresses of night work.

Summary

We do not yet know enough about the effects of shift work to make precise assessments of who will or will not be able to cope with the many varieties of shift systems. Moreover, we do not yet have a shift work selection tool that avoids making it blatantly obvious what response candidates should give according to whether or not they want a shift work position. It is more helpful, therefore, for shift-working nurses to think in terms of self-assessment, counseling, and education in order to promote shift work coping strategies. Since some individuals are more likely than others to have problems with circadian system adaptation and night performance, they should be warned about this before embarking on a shift work career. Interventions to facilitate shift work adaptation should be based on the nurse's individual goals and self-assessment of personal strengths and weaknesses related to shift work. The nurse's level of commitment to a particular shift system and position are important factors in determining how well he or she will adjust to shift work.

FIGURE 7.1
Sleep Diary

Month / Day of Week	A.M.	12:00–12:30	12:30–1:00	1:00–1:30	1:30–2:00	2:00–2:30	2:30–3:00	3:00–3:30	3:30–4:00	4:00–4:30	4:30–5:00	5:00–5:30	5:30–6:00	6:00–6:30	6:30–7:00	7:00–7:30	7:30–8:00	8:00–8:30	8:30–9:00	9:00–9:30	9:30–10:00	10:00–10:30	10:30–11:00	11:00–11:30	11:30–12:00
1																										
2																										
3																										
4																										
5																										
6																										
7																										
8																										
9																										
10																										
11																										
12																										
13																										
14																										
15																										
16																										
17																										
18																										
19																										
20																										
21																										
22																										
23																										
24																										
25																										
26																										
27																										
28																										
29																										
30																										
31																										

Instructions: Place a check in every box for each half hour you slept. Include all naps.

FIGURE 7.1 (continued)

P.M.	12:00–12:30	12:30– 1:00	1:00– 1:30	1:30– 2:00	2:00– 2:30	2:30– 3:00	3:00– 3:30	3:30– 4:00	4:00– 4:30	4:30– 5:00	5:00– 5:30	5:30– 6:00	6:00– 6:30	6:30– 7:00	7:00– 7:30	7:30– 8:00	8:00– 8:30	8:30– 9:00	9:00– 9:30	9:30–10:00	10:00–10:30	10:30–11:00	11:00–11:30	11:30–12:00	Hours worked

Instructions: Place a check in every box for each half hour you slept. Include all naps.

FIGURE 7.2
Sleep Quality Questionnaire

MAIN SLEEP PERIOD

1. Date: _____

2. Total hours of sleep today: _____

    From ____ a.m./p.m. to ____ a.m./p.m.

3. How long did it take you to fall asleep? _____

4. a) How many times do you remember waking up during the sleep
    period? _____

    b) Reasons for waking up: _____

5. a) How many times did you get up during the sleep period? _____

    b) Reasons for getting up:

    ____ Bathroom

    ____ Medication (type: _____)

    ____ Food/drink (type: _____)

    ____ Telephone

    ____ Doorbell

    ____ Other (describe: _____)

6. Was your sleep interrupted by any of the following?

    ____ Noise (# of times: ____)

    ____ Telephone (# of times: ____)

    ____ Visitors (# of times: ____)

    ____ Family (# of times: ____)

    ____ Other (describe: _____)

    ____ Sleep was not interrupted

7. Did you use an alarm clock to awaken? ____ Yes ____ No

8. Did someone else awaken you? ____ Yes ____ No

9. Did you wake up naturally? ____ Yes ____ No

FIGURE 7.2 (continued)

10. How was your sleep quality?

    ____ Very good   ____ Fair   ____ Very poor

    ____ Good   ____ Poor

11. How was your mood upon awakening?

    ____ Very good   ____ Fair   ____ Very poor

    ____ Good   ____ Poor

12. If you worked a night shift after a day's sleep:

    a) How sleepy were you during the night?

    ____ Not at all

    ____ Moderately

    ____ Extremely

    b) How tired were you when the shift ended?

    ____ Not at all

    ____ Moderately

    ____ Extremely

    c) Were you sleepy on the drive home? ____ Yes ____ No

NAPS

1. a) Did you take any naps in addition to your main period of sleep today?

    ____ Yes ____ No

    b) How many?___ [Please include naps taken during working hours, and mark them with an asterisk(*) below.]

    From ____ a.m./p.m. to ____ a.m./p.m.

    From ____ a.m./p.m. to ____ a.m./p.m.

    From ____ a.m./p.m. to ____ a.m./p.m.

FIGURE 7.3
Circadian Type Questionnaire (U)*

This questionnaire refers to your daily habits. For each question, indicate what you <u>prefer</u> to do or <u>can</u> do, not what you are <u>forced</u> to do by your present work schedule or routine. Work as quickly as possible, recording your immediate reaction to each question. There are no right or wrong answers. For each question, indicate where you fall between the two extremes given by drawing a short vertical line through the horizontal line printed below the question.

For example, if the question is:

Are you the sort of person who prefers to do their work in the morning?

| Definitely | Definitely not |

then a vertical mark placed as shown above would indicate a very strong preference for working in the morning. However, if you placed the mark as shown below:

| Definitely | Definitely not |

then it would indicate a complete indifference toward working in the morning. Similarly, degrees of dislike for working in the morning would be indicated by marking to the right of the center.

---

1. How easy do you find it to take short "cat naps" during the day?

   | Very easy | Very difficult |

2. If you have been out very late at a party, how easy do you find it to "sleep in" the following morning if there is nothing to prevent you from doing so?

   | Very difficult | Very easy |

3. If you have very little sleep one night, do you feel drowsy the following day?

   | Very much so | Hardly at all |

4. If you are awakened at an unusual time, can you "wake up" properly and do whatever it is you have to do?

   | Only with great difficulty | Very easily |

5. To what extent are you better at working at certain times of the day or night than at others?

   | No difference | Very much so |

*From S. Folkard, T.H. Monk, and M.C. Lobban, 1979, "Towards a Predictive Test of Adjustment to Shiftwork," *Ergonomics* 22:79-91.

FIGURE 7.3 (continued)

6. Do you ever get a "second wind" if you stay up very late?

_____
Never   Always

7. If you have something important to do but feel very drowsy, can you overcome your drowsiness?

_____
Only with great difficulty   Very easily

8. Do you go to bed at a fixed time and get up at a fixed time, even if you don't have to?

_____
Never   Always

9. After you have had several late nights in a row, how easy do you find it to get to sleep if you go to bed early to try to "catch up"?

_____
Very easily   Very difficult

10. Do you have episodes (several nights in a row) when you find it difficult to get to sleep?

_____
Seldom   Frequently

11. To what extent do you prefer to have your meals at fixed times?

_____
No preference   Strong preference

12. If you have an alcoholic drink at lunchtime, does it affect you more than the same drink would in the evening? (Please omit this question if you do not drink.)

_____
A lot more   No difference

13. How do you react to working at unusual times of the day or night?

_____
Dislike it a lot   Enjoy it a lot

14. Are you the sort of person who can easily skip a night's sleep?

_____
Definitely not   Definitely

FIGURE 7.3 (continued)

15. How easy do you find it to sleep during the day if you have to?

_____

Very difficult   Very easy

16. When you are away on vacation, to what extent do you stick to your normal times of getting up and going to bed?

_____

Very different   Exactly the same

17. If you don't have an alarm clock, can you successfully "tell yourself" to wake up at a certain time?

_____

Always   Never

18. Do you find it easy to get up very early in the morning if, for example, you are leaving for a trip?

_____

Very difficult   Very easy

19. Are you the sort of person who feels far livelier during the day than early in the morning or late at night?

_____

Definitely not   Definitely

20. When you have had to get up at the same time for several days in a row, do you start waking up just before your alarm clock goes off?

_____

Never   Frequently

FIGURE 7.3 (continued)
Computing Your Circadian Type Score

After completing the Circadian Type Questionnaire, compute your rigidity-of-sleep habits (Rs) score, your vigor (V) score, and your morningness (M) score as follows:

For each question, measure (in millimeters) from the beginning point (left-hand side) of the horizontal line to the vertical point you marked on the line. Record your measurement in the appropriate place on the score sheet. The scoring scale is 0-99. [Please note that the answer to question 12 is not included in the scoring.]

Rigidity-of-Sleep (Rs) Score

For your Rs score, total your answers to questions 1, 8, 9, 10, 11, and 16. That total is sum 1. Then add up your answers to questions 2 and 15. That total is sum 2. To find sum 3, subtract sum 2 from 198. Finally, add sum 1 and sum 3 and divide that total by 8. Round that quotient to the nearest whole number, and you've got your Rs score. The higher your Rs score, the less flexible you are about your sleep habits.

Vigor (V) Score

For your V score, total your answers to questions 3, 4, 7, and 14 to arrive at sum 1. Use your answer to question 5 as sum 2, then subtract sum 2 from 99 to find sum 3. Add sum 1 and sum 3 and divide the total by 5. Round off the quotient to the nearest whole number and you have your V score. The lower your V score, the less able you are to overcome drowsiness.

Morningness (M) Score

For your M score, total your answers to questions 18, 19, and 20 for sum 1. Total your answers to questions 6, 13, and 17 for sum 2. Subtract sum 2 from 297 for sum 3. Add sum 1 and sum 3, divide the total by 6, round the quotient off to the nearest whole number, and you have your M score. The higher your M score, the more you are a morning type. The lower your M score, the more you are an evening type.

FIGURE 7.3 (continued)
Circadian Type Questionnaire Score Sheet

Write your millimeter measures next to the question numbers, then follow the directions from the previous page to find your total scores.

Example

Vigor (V) score:

Question 3 _74_
Question 4 _77_
Question 7 _83_
Question 14 _98_
Sum 1 = _332_
Question 5 = sum 2 = _66_
99 − sum 2 = sum 3 = _33_
Sum 1 + sum 3 = _365_ ÷ 5 = V score = | _73_ |

Rigidity-of-Sleep (Rs) Score
Question 1 ____
Question 8 ____
Question 9 ____
Question 10 ____
Question 11 ____
Question 16 ____
Sum 1 = ____
Question 2 ____
Question 15 ____
Sum 2 = ____
198 − sum 2 = sum 3 = ____
Sum 1 + sum 3 = ____ ÷ 8 = Rs score = | |

Vigor (V) Score
Question 3 ____
Question 4 ____
Question 7 ____
Question 14 ____
Sum 1 = ____
Question 5 = sum 2 = ____
99 − sum 2 = sum 3 = ____
Sum 1 + sum 3 = ____ ÷ 5 = V score = | |

Morningness (M) Score
Question 18 ____
Question 19 ____
Question 20 ____
Sum 1 = ____
Question 6 ____
Question 13 ____
Question 17 ____
Sum 2 = ____
297 − sum 2 = sum 3 = ____
Sum 1 + sum 3 = ____ ÷ 6 = M score = | |

— Chapter 8 —

Nurses' Shift Work
Awareness Program

Introduction

Adequately coping with shift work is not merely a matter of getting enough sleep (see Chapters 2 and 3). The shift-working nurse's sleep, biological clock, and social and domestic requirements must be viewed as an integrated whole — each of these factors affects the others and, ultimately, the nurse's shift work coping ability. For example, if you are not getting enough sleep, you will start taking naps at inappropriate times of day, which will upset your biological clock, cause you to become anxious and irritable, and eventually create tension between you and your family. Since sleep, biological clock, and social and domestic needs are so interrelated, any shift work awareness program has to involve a "whole life" approach — becoming a natural part of the nurse's work <u>and</u> home lives; it cannot be just an "at work" approach. Figure 8.1 illustrates how sleep, biological clock, and social/domestic factors interrelate and work together to influence how well a nurse copes with shift work.

The next section of this chapter will provide background information necessary to create effective personal goals for a Nurses' Shift Work Awareness Program (NSWAP). The purpose of the NSWAP is to develop strategies geared toward restoring balance to sleep, biological, and social/domestic factors. The "Implementing

Shift Work Coping Strategies" section will present specific strategies that should be helpful to your particular shift work situation.

Shift Work Coping Strategies: An Integrated Whole

Sleep Factors

In addition to the detailed background on sleep presented in Chapter 5, the important thing to remember about sleep with regard to developing an NSWAP is that it has both rhythmic and homeostatic attributes. Just as how hungry we feel depends both on whether it is a mealtime (a rhythmic attribute) and how long it has been since we last ate (a homeostatic attribute), so too is sleep dependent on these attributes. Sleep also is both a circadian rhythm in its own right, as well as a time cue, or zeitgeber, for other circadian rhythms. Moreover, by its very nature, the rhythm of sleep controls exposure to other powerful zeitgebers, such as light. The major sleep episode inevitably plunges us into several hours of subjective darkness and relative immobility. While chronobiologists may argue about the relative strengths of various zeitgebers, none would dispute that the sleep-wake cycle constitutes a very powerful circadian time cue. Shift-working nurses should be aware of this, and should incorporate the timing of sleep into their NSWAP strategies.

In addition to the rhythmic influence of sleep, there also is the homeostatic aspect of sleep, which varies as a function of how long it has been since sleep last occurred. This relationship has been outlined in a mathematical model of the human circadian system, which proposes a "Process S" that builds up during wakefulness and dissipates during slow wave sleep (Borbély, 1982). The timing of sleep onset is then controlled by a combination of the status of the circadian clock (as indicated, for example, by the body temperature rhythm) and the amount of Process S that has built up. Thus, this pressure can sometimes be used to help induce sleep when needed. A "grazing" attitude toward sleep (taking lots of naps) should be avoided, as it can take the edge off Process S buildup, thereby making a consolidated episode of sleep more difficult to obtain.

Biological Clock Factors

Your biological clock is located deep inside your brain (see Chapter 2). The function of the biological clock is to prepare your body and mind for sleep at certain times of the day, and for activity at other times. Unfortunately for the shift worker, the clock is slow to change after a disruption in routine. Until it completes that change, the shift worker's biological clock will be expecting sleep at the wrong time of day and, therefore, shutting down functions (like alertness and appetite) that should still be active, and also activating those functions and causing wakefulness when the shift worker is attempting to sleep.

Since the biological clock is located inside the brain, it has no direct way of differentiating "night" from "day" — it can only function on the information it is given. In developing NSWAP strategies, this information can be manipulated using zeitgebers to improve the chances of getting the desired biological clock effect. Zeitgeber management, therefore, is an integral part of the circadian component of any NSWAP. Shift-working nurses need to know which zeitgebers are positive (working in favor of biological clock adjustment) and which are negative (working against adjustment) in order to successfully adjust their biological clocks to expect new hours of sleep and wakefulness. These distinctions are discussed later in this chapter.

Nurse shift workers also need to know which time cues are strong and which ones are comparatively weak and ineffectual. Through the 1970s, most experts agreed that the cycle of daylight and darkness was not a very important time cue for human beings (Wever, 1979). In 1980, however, attention became focused on a pineal hormone in the blood called *melatonin,* which is associated with sleepiness when circulating in the bloodstream, and which seems to be an important part of the biological clock. Peak plasma levels of melatonin usually occur at night, but that peak can be eliminated by placing the subject (with eyes open) in extremely bright light. Surprisingly, however, this effect does not occur under artificial illumination from <u>ordinary</u> electric ceiling lights (Lewy et al., 1980). It seems, therefore, that <u>daylight</u> illumination levels might play a special role as time cues, being particularly effective at resetting the biological clock. Unfortunately, this is bad news for the shift-working nurse, who has no control over sunrise and sunset. Therefore, some experts recommend the use of extremely bright lights to simulate daylight. Although these "light boxes" have been shown to work well in the laboratory (Czeisler et al., 1990) and with astronauts (Czeisler, Chiasera, and Duffy, 1991), they often are very difficult to install in ordinary workplaces, and are almost impossible in most hospital units (since they would keep patients awake). Moreover, even when light boxes are installed in a nurse's home, the time constraints of a shift work schedule often limit his or her ability to sit in front of the lights for the recommended three hours a day.

In addition to daylight, many other factors also function as zeitgebers. Patterns of eating and sleeping, noise and temperature levels, and simple social contacts have all been shown to be zeitgebers (Wever, 1979). In the following section, we will outline strategies that use these time cues in order to help nurse shift workers obtain the biological clock changes they want.

Social/Domestic Factors

As mentioned earlier in this chapter, a nurse's home life can be a very powerful force in affecting the amount of sleep obtained and the sort of behavior patterns that have a direct impact on the biological clock. In an unpublished shift work study conducted by Dr. Monk in 1982, one shift worker's home environment had become so unbearable that he spent most of his sleep periods in his car. Clearly, advice about "time cues" and "good sleep habits" would not have been of much help until the shift worker's domestic problems were resolved.

A nurse shift worker's first social/domestic strategy, therefore, must be to provide the sort of environment in which sleep and biological clock goals can be obtained. Secondly, domestic issues like parenting difficulties, social demands, and spousal communication problems also will require close attention so as not to affect the shift worker's biological clock. Therefore, a nurse shift worker must develop effective methods of communication, time management, and domestic task definition in order to ensure that:

- family members and close friends understand the shift work schedule and related problems;
- sleep, family interaction, and social activities all receive regular attention; and
- all domestic responsibilities are shared and completed on a regular basis.

Although many shift workers and their families will regard these strategies as inconvenient and time-consuming, the rewards of implementing such a plan (e.g., avoiding a divorce) undoubtedly will far outweigh any potential aggravation.

Implementing Shift Work Coping Strategies

After all of the shift work background information presented in the first seven chapters of this book, the specific shift work coping strategies outlined in this chapter should not seem too surprising. We have organized this book around a solid core of background information about shift work and the biological clock because we believe that if nurses can understand a specific coping strategy within an overall framework of the dynamics of shift work, then they are much more likely to incorporate that strategy into their lifestyles and to stick with it. Also, through understanding general information about shift work coping strategies, nurse shift workers will be able to develop alternate strategies if their work situations change (from fixed to rotating shifts, for example).

The following section is divided into strategies concerned with sleep, biological clock, and social/domestic factors.

Sleep Factors

Sleep is as important to you as oxygen — treat it that way! Do not let social or work pressures interfere with your sleeptime. If you find yourself spending most of your days off catching up on sleep, you are not getting enough during the week. It is okay to get an extra hour or two of sleep on days off — feeling the need for more than that can indicate that you are getting "overdrawn" in your sleep "bank account." Since sleep is most refreshing when it is not interrupted, napping should only be regarded as an emergency "fill up," and not as an integral part of your sleep strategy.

Unless you are sick or chronically sleep-deprived, it is not possible to get a good amount of refreshing sleep totally at will — your body and mind both have to be ready for sleep. Regular sleep habits will help diminish the feeling of needing more sleep, so try to stick to a consistent bedtime as much as possible, even on your days off. A correctly set biological clock is the single most important factor in assuring you good sleep with few jet-lag-type effects.

Set the stage for your sleep period by darkening the bedroom with heavy shades, blinds, or shutters; going through all the same pre-bed rituals you would for a night sleep (brushing your teeth, putting on pajamas, etc.); and disconnecting the telephone and doorbell. Put a sign on your bedroom door that says, "Shift Worker Asleep!" This is your sleeptime — do not let anyone or anything disrupt it.

Keep your bedroom as a haven for sleep. Do your bill paying, TV watching, and ironing in other rooms. If you start to do too many varied activities in the bedroom, you will begin to associate the bedroom with stress rather than relaxation.

Get your body ready for sleep. Since caffeine remains in your bloodstream for up to five hours, do not drink any caffeinated beverage within five hours of your expected bedtime, or it will keep you awake when you are trying to sleep. Also avoid the trap of using alcohol to put yourself to sleep. Although alcohol will put you to sleep, getting to sleep is not the problem for most shift workers. Staying asleep and getting the right sort of sleep are the problems, and alcohol makes both of these a lot more difficult (Buysse, 1991).

As discussed in Chapter 5, not only is the amount of sleep you get important, but so is the type of sleep. Your goal should be to get plenty of deep, refreshing slow wave sleep, and to avoid too much REM sleep. Eating lightly, avoiding caffeine and alcohol, and drinking warm milk before bedtime are likely to increase slow wave sleep.

Although the last seven chapters have presented many good reasons why a shift-working nurse might not sleep well, many nurses might still believe that their sleep problems indicate an illness requiring medical treatment. If you sleep well on vacations, however, your poor day sleeps after night work are unlikely to indicate an illness. While there may be something wrong with what you are doing with regard to routines, time cues, meals, and sleep patterns, there is probably nothing medically wrong. It is perfectly natural to find it difficult to sleep during the day — we are built that way! This perception of illness has caused many shift workers to seek medical advice and to be treated with hypnotics, which initially might seem like a worthwhile strategy. When sleeping pills are first used, they do help you get some decent sleep. What they will not do, however, is reset the biological clock; when they are stopped, therefore, you are still left with disrupted sleep. This fact was presented in a study in which night shift workers were given either triazolam (0.5 mg.) or a placebo on the first two days of sleep, and then received only a placebo on the next two days of sleep. Although the drug aided sleep on the days it was given, no further advantages were gained from the drug. The shift workers' circadian systems had not generally benefitted from the two good days of sleep, or from the hypnotic that allowed them (Walsh, Muehlbach, and Schweitzer, 1984).

The real dangers of hypnotics are *tolerance* (when the drug stops having any helpful effect) and *dependence* (when withdrawal effects occur upon attempting to quit the drug). The effects of tolerance and dependence can give the impression that the hypnotics are actually doing some good when, in fact, they may have long ago lost the power to provide any genuine relief. Moreover, chronic use of some sleeping pills can lead to irritability and/or drowsiness — just the sort of problems that shift-working nurses do not need to add to their lives.

The occasional use of sleeping pills to get over a particularly bad sleeping spell can be helpful. Anyone using sleeping pills on a regular basis, however (more than three times per week), would be strongly advised to begin tapering off the drug. You might lose a bit of sleep during the tapering-off process, but it will greatly benefit your health in the long run, and will not stop you from being able to use sleeping pills occasionally in the future. Indeed, tapering off from regular use will make future occasional use of hypnotics much more effective.

Biological Clock Factors

In order to set tangible goals for your biological clock, you have to know in which direction and by what amount you want to reset it. Except for some very rapidly rotating shift systems (such as a cycle of two mornings-two evenings-two nights-two days off, or two or three 12-hour night shifts in a row), most shift systems require as rapid a resetting of the biological clock as possible. (We will discuss very rapidly rotating shift systems later in this section.)

For purposes of the following discussion, we will assume that you want to reset your biological clock to become appropriate to your new work/sleep routine as rapidly as possible, and to keep it at that orientation for as long as you work that particular shift.

Let us first consider night shifts, which usually require the biggest circadian changes. For night shift work, what you typically try to do is get the biological clock to expect work from 11:00 p.m./12:00 a.m. to 7:00/8:00 a.m., and sleep from 8:00/9:00 a.m. to about 4:00 p.m. Note that this is not an exact schedule inversion; rather, it is a schedule delay by about nine hours. Instead of going to bed at midnight, you would go to bed at 9:00 a.m., waking up (ideally) at 4:00 p.m. rather than 7:00 a.m. This is important to know because the biological clock copes more easily with delays in routine than with advances (see Chapter 2); adjustment to a six-hour advance can take just as long as adjustment to a nine-hour delay. Therefore, delay changes in routine are certainly the best choice whenever possible.

In order to assist this phase delay process, it is important to <u>go to bed as soon as possible after your night shift</u>. Get home as quickly as possible, have a light meal and a warm milk drink, and go straight to bed. Avoid the temptation to do domestic chores first. The earlier you can get to bed, the fewer adjustments your biological clock will have to make, the fewer sleep interruptions you will experience, and the fewer jet-lag-type symptoms you will feel. Only use naps before going on shift as a "topping out" measure, and keep them to two hours or less. Otherwise, imagine the confusion your biological clock will go through trying to figure out which sleep episode is supposed to be the "night" sleep.

Sleep episodes, however, are not the only time cue on which your biological clock depends. As mentioned earlier in this chapter, daylight also may be a strong time cue. Therefore, as strange as it may sound, it might be helpful to <u>wear dark sunglasses on your drive home from work</u>, especially if you live to the east of your place of work and find yourself driving home toward the sun. Wearing sunglasses will make it more difficult for your melatonin surge to be suppressed, and for your biological clock to thus lose its delayed phase.

Other time cues your biological clock will be paying attention to are meal timings and other aspects of your daily routine. <u>Try to eat three balanced meals a day</u>, and try to keep them at regular times as much as possible. Initiate or continue a physical fitness program with as much regularity as you can manage. <u>Everything you can do to regulate your routine will help your biological clock recognize when you want it to be "day" and when you want it to be "night."</u>

Let us imagine that you have followed all of this advice and now find yourself with two days off at the end of a week of night shifts. With regard to sleep, what should you do now? The answer depends on whether you are on a rotating shift and will be switching to morning or evening shifts after the break, or whether you are working fixed shifts and will be continuing with night shifts after the break.

If you are changing shifts after the break, your goal will be to reset your biological clock toward nighttime sleep. Therefore, it is best to have a <u>short</u> (two hours or less) nap after the last night shift of the week, and then allow yourself good long <u>night</u> sleeps on your days off. This sleep schedule is also best from a social and domestic point of view, especially if you have children at home. The advantage of this sleep schedule is that all the powerful time cues that were working against you on the night shift are now working in your favor to rapidly reestablish a day-active orientation for your circadian system.

A very different approach has to be taken if you are on a fixed night or slowly rotating shift system. In this case, you will want to retain as much of your biological clock's night-active orientation as you possibly can. For shift workers with families and/or social commitments, however, it is often difficult to stick to a nocturnal schedule. As a compromise, therefore, you should get up as late as possible in the morning and go to bed as late as possible at night; wear dark sunglasses or stay indoors during the morning; and try to stick to as much of your meal and exercise schedules as possible. This approach is not easy, and most of us lose a lot of our biological clock's night-active orientation during days off; however, these strategies can help lessen the shift work burden.

A shift system that has become very popular in Europe is the *very rapid rotation system,* in which no more than two or three night shifts are ever worked in a row. A typical shift example is the "continental" or "metropolitan" rotation schedule of two mornings-two evenings-two nights-two days off (the 2-2-2 system). Other rapid rotation shift schedules compress the work week into three 12-hour shifts. The advantage of very rapid rotation is that the biological clock does not have time to change; therefore, there are no long-term jet-lag-type effects, fewer stomach problems, etc. Not changing the biological clock, however, can also create problems. For instance, the day sleeps in-between the night shifts are severely disrupted because the biological clock is totally day-active oriented; night shift alertness and performance can suffer for the same reason. Even so, many shift workers do prefer rapid rotation systems because there is not enough time on the night shift to build up too much of a "sleep debt." Additionally, keeping a day-active orientation to the biological clock, and thereby lessening scheduling problems during days off, is an attractive schedule to most shift workers. Rapid rotation works particularly well when the job demands a lot of thinking or activity and keeps you too busy to feel sleepy during the night shifts (such as critical care or perioperative nursing). Strategies for coping with a rapidly rotating system need to be very different from those for more slowly rotating or fixed shifts. For rapid rotation, the key is to retain a day-active orientation to the circadian system. Exposure to daylight should be maximized, and a regular day-active routine of meals and exercise should be maintained as much as possible.

Generally, in thinking about implementing your own biological clock strategies, try to imagine yourself as your biological clock, located deep inside your head. You know when the body eats, lays down to sleep, and exerts itself. You know when daylight is hitting the eyes and when things are loud or quiet. Just where you, as a biological clock, decide to put "night" and where to put "day" will depend only upon that mixture of information. The more consistent that information is and the more regular it is over time, the easier and quicker will be the final decision and readjustment.

Social/Domestic Factors

Ideally, we would like the families and roommates of shift-working nurses to be just as involved in understanding and implementing the information presented in this book as the nurses themselves. Social and domestic problems related to shift work affect everyone in the shift worker's family (see Chapter 3); solutions and strategies, therefore, also must come from the entire family.

Earlier in this chapter, we discussed the need for the shift worker to maintain regular sleeptime and waketime routines, as well as the three recommended ways to enhance social/domestic coping strategies:

1) developing patterns of communication,
2) managing time, and
3) defining domestic tasks.

These strategies will involve considerable effort by all household members, will restrict them from making noise and demands on the shift worker's time, and will sometimes involve spending money to implement specific strategies. These activities may seem unpleasant, but remember that they are geared toward maintaining positive and effective family relationships.

To protect yourself from the noise of household activity during your sleep period, you may need to make some purchases. You will need heavy drapes or blinds to cut out light in the bedroom, a set of good earplugs (cotton balls do not work!), and maybe some rugs or carpeting to help deaden sound. An air conditioner or fan for the bedroom can also help muffle outside noises (and will make sleeping less uncomfortable during the summer). Headphones for televisions, radios, and stereos enable other family members to listen to music or watch TV programs without disturbing your sleep. Additionally, a VCR will allow you to watch any TV program when <u>you</u> like. In very noisy neighborhoods, it might even be worth investing in an "ocean waves" sound machine to camouflage outside noises and help you relax. If necessary, replace your telephones with the type that allow you to totally turn off the ringer, get a telephone answering machine, and install a switch on the doorbell so that you can disconnect it while sleeping. <u>If the only person at home is a shift-working nurse trying to sleep, there effectively is no one at home</u>!

Define your sleeptimes and stick to them. Ignore deliveries, reschedule appointments and shopping when possible, and warn friends not to call during your sleeptime. Although these efforts will not always guarantee uninterrupted sleep, they usually will ensure some improvement in your sleep. All household members should make every effort to avoid forcing the shift-working nurse to shorten or alter the timing of his or her sleep. If everyone in the household knows when the shift worker's sleeptime is, the strategies are much easier to enforce. During the shift worker's sleeptime, make it a family rule that headphones are enforced, vacuum cleaning is banned, and the phones and doorbells are silenced. Family members will soon realize that, despite the extra effort involved, a well-rested shift worker is much more agreeable to live with than a tired one!

Communication with friends and family members is very important. Place a large monthly planning calendar in the kitchen, and highlight the days of each month when you will be working days, evenings, or nights. During night shifts, tack up a note reminding the family of the "quiet times" when you will be trying to sleep. The more family members and friends know about your work schedule and sleeptimes, the less likely they will be to thoughtlessly create problems for you. Make friends with other shift-working families; they will understand and be more sensitive to your pressures and limitations. Talk to your family about the things that are annoying you at work. Tell them when you are upset because of your shift work schedule, and when you are upset because of something they have or have not done. <u>If your anger is because of your shift work, blame the shift work — do not take it out on your family</u>!

Reserving time for various social activities also will help your shift work adjustment process. In addition to setting aside time for sleep, it also is very important to set aside time for your children, your spouse, and your friends. <u>Remember that these activities are so much more important than domestic chores or shopping</u>. Of course, domestic tasks have to be done, and time should be set aside for them, but do not let these tasks interfere with the time you need to spend with your family or the time you need to sleep. Family members can be of tremendous help in completing household chores, especially (as is so often the case) when the shift-working nurse is also expected to be a homemaker. Define and assign chores, set the times by which they must be completed, and <u>everyone</u> will benefit.

As we have stated repeatedly, shift work can be a major source of stress, which can be either invigorating or destructive. If a family is to cope successfully with shift work, it must recognize the inherent stresses and create productive ways to deal with them. By committing itself to working together to cope with shift work, a nurse shift worker's family can only grow in cohesiveness and strength.

Staying Alert

No matter how well you follow the advice given in this book, there inevitably will be times during or after your shift when keeping alert becomes a significant problem. Although caffeine may be of some help, there also are behavioral strategies to help you to stay awake. For instance, varying your task routines at work, walking or stretching every 30 minutes or so, and giving yourself mini-rewards (e.g., a snack break halfway through your shift) can all help make your shift pass more quickly and with fewer lulls in alertness. Depending on the safety of your work neighborhood, a stroll in the fresh air might help, too. For the benefit of regulating your biological clock, however, it is best not to nap during shift breaks; instead, try to create social opportunities on your breaks (lively conversation will help keep you awake). In general, varying your shift routine as much as possible can be a real asset in helping you stay alert.

Additionally, no NSWAP would be complete without a serious caveat regarding the drive home after an evening or a night shift. Arguably, this might be the most dangerous activity a shift-working nurse undertakes. Many of the nurses we spoke with for this book reported having accidents or near-misses on past drives home from work.

Evening shift nurses are in triple jeopardy when it comes to driving risks. First, they are tired, and their bodies are starting to shut down various functions in anticipation of sleep. Second, it is dark, and traffic accidents are more likely to occur in darkness than in daylight. Third, many of the people they are sharing the road with are likely to be intoxicated. Evening shift nurses should drive very defensively on the way home, regarding every other driver as a potential drunk, giving them a wide berth, and anticipating erratic driving behavior. For the night shift nurse, it is daylight during the drive home, and there are usually fewer drunk drivers on the roads. The night shift nurse's fatigue level, however, is likely to be more intense than that of an evening shift nurse.

Staying alert on the drive home from work is critical for all shift-working nurses. The car interior should be kept cool, with some lively music or conversation on the radio to keep you from nodding off. If you have a citizens band radio, use it to talk with other drivers, or carpool to work so you will have someone to keep you company. Varying your route to and from work, and making a point of noticing things along the way (a new restaurant or a building's construction process), can be effective ways of diverting fatigue while driving. Dr. Monk used to sing (rather badly!) at the top of his voice to help him stay awake. These strategies may seem like small things, but they might become lifesavers some day!

We do _not_ recommend stopping off for a late-night drink to "unwind." Besides eventually posing a safety hazard to yourself and other drivers on the road, drinking on the way home from work is not a good idea because it will make changes in your biological clock's timing more difficult to adjust to. If you get to bed at 1:30 a.m., for instance, all you have to contend with is a couple of hours difference from a normal day sleep. If you spend a couple of extra hours in a bar, however, you have effectively become a night shift worker — not getting to bed until almost dawn. Additionally, although alcohol can help you _fall_ asleep, it makes staying asleep more difficult, and changes your level of sleep to one that is less refreshing. Instead of a nightcap, it is much better to unwind from work with a light snack or milk drink at home, and then <u>get to bed early</u>.

Summary

The information presented in this chapter is not intended to offer magic solutions for your shift work problems. Shift work problems are multifaceted, and require multifaceted solutions — there are no easy answers. Rather, we hope to have provided you with a wide variety of strategies, based on sound scientific principles, that you can adapt to your own personal circumstances in order to successfully cope with shift work.

FIGURE 8.1

Factors Affecting Shift Work Coping Ability

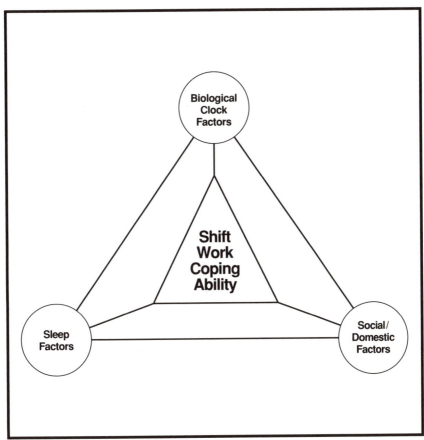

From Monk, 1988.

Chapter 9

The Nurse Administrator's Role

Introduction

After presenting background material on the circadian system, shift work self-assessment, and shift work coping strategies in the preceding chapters, we now turn to the role of nurse executives, managers, educators, and researchers in shift systems. (For convenience in this chapter, we will often use the term "nurse administrator" to represent all of these nurses.) Since some of the interventions that can increase shift work coping and adjustment are beyond the direct control of nurse shift workers, nurse administrators can be of great assistance in improving shift systems and, subsequently, the well-being of nurse shift workers and their patients. Nurse administrators have direct input into the types and hours of shifts, the scheduling of meal services, and the timing of inservice education programs — all of which should be made convenient for shift workers.

Ignoring shift work issues can be costly in terms of patient liability and nursing personnel management issues. All too frequently, the connection between shift work and resulting costs is not made. A high number of nighttime falls, medication errors, and other patient incidents; high turnover and absenteeism rates; low recruitment rates; high vacancy rates; and other quality control and personnel issues may be related to shift work concerns that have not been adequately addressed by nurse executives. As the costs of recruiting, orienting, and retaining nurses continue to increase, nurse executives cannot afford to overlook the large and valuable number of nurses who work evening and night shifts on a regular or occasional basis.

We wish there was more evidence that the nursing profession is using published research results concerning performance, physiological and psychological rhythms, adaptability, and the well-being of shift workers to improve shift systems and provide support for nurse shift workers. Shift rotation and night shift coverage policies vary, all too often, according to management philosophies and the availability of permanent night shift nurses. Educational and support services that foster informed shift selection and adaptability are rare. Nurse shift workers might feel that they are being ignored by nurse administrators, especially if the administrators fail to make rounds or hold regular staff meetings with shift workers, or to offer in-service and continuing education programs at convenient times for evening and night shift nurses.

On the positive side, however, we must point out that nurse administrators, particularly in urban hospitals, have been found to be more innovative in developing shift rotation methods than executives in some other industries. Comparing the shift work characteristics of nurses with those of emergency medical technicians, airline customer service representatives, police officers, and telephone operators, one study investigated compensation, control over scheduling, and periodicity and patterning of scheduling (McLaughlin and Mohr, 1988). In all three areas, nursing offered a greater variety of shift work options than did the other four groups of workers. Nursing was the only group with any evidence of self-scheduling, was the most flexible in terms of patterning and scheduling options, and had shift differentials that equaled or exceeded those of the other groups.

Types of Shift Systems

Shift systems have been studied by chronobiologists and chronopsychologists in order to identify a system that is most acceptable to the greatest number of employers and shift workers from physiological, psychological, and social perspectives. Much of this literature reports studies of patterns widely used in European industries by male shift workers. Although there are no known descriptive data on the numbers and types of shift systems presently used in the wide range of nursing service settings, it is known that many nurse administrators use rotating shift workers to supplement the ranks of voluntary permanent evening and night shift nurses. Involuntary assignment to permanent evening and night shifts does occur, although much less frequently. When shift rotation is required, nurses generally rotate between day shifts and either evening or night shifts; they are not commonly assigned to all three shifts in one week. Rigid rotation patterns are used infrequently. Many hospitals rotate nurses on a weekly schedule. In a limited number of health care institutions, no permanent night shift nurses are employed for philosophical reasons; in others, there are no rotating shift nurses except in cases of unscheduled absences or emergencies. Several nurse executives told us they prefer shift rotation so that all staff nurses are exposed to the complete patient care continuum. Others had reservations about the isolation and competence of permanent night shift workers.

For most nurse administrators who deal with shift workers, the primary concern is whether the best possible form of shift system is in place. As we have pointed out in earlier chapters, that concern, unfortunately, is not always easily addressed with a "cookbook" answer. Before determining whether a particular shift system is best, it is necessary for nurse administrators to first explore the advantages and disadvantages of several shift options.

Permanent Shifts

In general, permanent and slowly rotating shift patterns are more common in the United States than in other industrialized nations, where there is a clear trend toward rapidly rotating shift systems (Kogi, 1985). Early investigators realized that the well-being of shift workers depends upon maintaining the synchronization of all circadian rhythms, and that shift systems should be designed to minimize the effects of conflicting zeitgebers on the timing of these rhythms. Many of these early researchers advocated permanent night shifts or rotations of at least one month, based on studies showing that the complete inversion and resynchronization of circadian rhythms was only very slowly achieved by many of the physiological variables after a phase change in the sleep-activity cycle (Kleitman, 1960; Teleky, 1943).

Later studies showed only partial inversion of some of the circadian rhythms after many consecutive nights of work, and a rapid reversion of the body temperature rhythm to its diurnal pattern when subjects slept at night, even as infrequently as once a week. Some forms of long-term circadian adjustment were seen in full-time permanent night shift workers when compared to part-time and rotating shift workers. Long-term adjustment is thought to be influenced by the worker's level of commitment to the shift system (Alward and Monk, 1990; Folkard, Monk, and Lobban, 1978).

Fixed shift assignment is an option that can work well in some circumstances. With fixed shifts, the nurse executive's chief problem usually is obtaining enough volunteers to cover the evening and night shifts. Solutions to this problem may include providing a greater financial incentive to work evenings or nights by improving the shift differential or paying a bonus, granting extra days off for evening or night work, or allowing seniority bidding in facilities with collective bargaining agreements. Some nursing shift system policies involve assigning newly-hired nurses to fixed evening or night shifts until there are day shift openings, which are then filled in order of seniority and interest. We suspect that retention is a problem when nurses are forced to work permanent evening or night shifts for long periods against their wishes, although we found no studies to substantiate this.

Advantages of a permanent night shift system stem from the probability that many permanent night shift nurses will gain and maintain a nocturnal orientation, while at the same time a high percentage of the nursing staff will be excused from shift rotation and its problems. There can be physiological, psychological, social, economic, and educational benefits for those nurses who find that permanent evening or night shifts best fit their professional and social needs. Additionally, patient care may benefit from the strong teamwork and continuity of care facilitated by permanent shift assignments.

Slow Shift Rotation

Many North American industries have opted to use slow shift rotation rather than permanent shift assignments. The more well-informed industries rotate workers in the direction of phase delays (days-to-evenings-to-nights) rather than phase advances (nights-to-evenings-to-days). As we discussed in Chapter 2, delays in routine to a later time of day are less difficult for biological clock adjustment than advances in routine to an earlier time of day.

Some industries have been successful with phase-delayed shift rotations every three weeks (Czeisler, Moore-Ede, and Coleman,

1982). This gives the biological clock three weeks to convert to a night-active orientation from the evening shift rotation, and to maintain the nocturnal adjustment before changing back to the day shift. The key issue in slow shift rotation patterns is to make certain that the nocturnal orientation is not lost on nonworking nights. It is by no means definite that a night-active orientation can be carried over those breaks unless the shift worker has a consistent nocturnal routine and limited exposure to competing time cues (such as a bright and noisy bedroom).

As the result of our interviews for this book, we agree with McLaughlin and Mohr's (1988) findings that slow rotation schedules are much less common in most nursing organizations than rotations of a week or less. We found no nursing organizations that used a rigid pattern of slow rotation through all three shifts; the majority of nurses are off duty every other weekend, and therefore have single days off in the middle of the week. Cyclical rotation patterns are used in some organizations, but more nursing departments now generate schedules through automated staffing and scheduling modules that are part of integrated nursing management systems.

Rapid Shift Rotation

Because of the difficulty most night workers have in trying to maintain a constant sleep-activity cycle and circadian system synchronization after more than a few night shifts, some European chronobiologists recommend rapid rotation rather than slow rotation or fixed shift schedules. With rapid rotation, no more than two or three night shifts are worked consecutively. A typical example is the European "continental" or "metropolitan" rotation of two days-two evenings-two nights-two days off (the 2-2-2 system). One of the few formal rapid shift rotation systems in the United States is the "rattler" used by some air traffic controllers, in which all three shifts are experienced within a given week. After workers overcome suspicion of the novelty of this shift system, their only major complaint usually involves having to keep up with their frequently changing work schedule. A modified form of rapid rotation involves rotating to a 12-hour night shift for up to three consecutive nights; however, the pattern is usually not rigid and the nurses rotate to two rather than three different shifts.

The advantage of rapid rotation is that the biological clock does not adjust to the phase changes, and symptoms of circadian dissociation are thus avoided. The disadvantage is that night shift alertness and performance can suffer on the shifts when nurses' circadian rhythms are geared toward sleep. Deficits in alertness and performance levels can be very dangerous for both patients and nurses, particularly if nurses are involved in fairly monotonous tasks that require high levels of vigilance, such as watching cardiac monitors or driving home from work. Another disadvantage of rapid shift rotation is that sleeping during the day is difficult for these unadjusted nurses.

The rapid rotation system works particularly well for night work involving highly cognitive skills, such as that required of professional nurses; research has demonstrated that phase shift adaptation may not benefit this type of performance (Folkard and Monk, 1979). If the position demands a significant amount of thinking or physical activity, the night nurse is often kept too busy to feel sleepy during the two night shifts.

Weekly Shift Rotation

Unfortunately, the shift system that is the most harmful to the circadian system is also one of the most common rotation systems throughout the United States — weekly shift rotation. In this type of shift system, workers have between four and seven days on a particular shift (days, evenings, or nights), and then a few days off before rotating to the next shift. Weekly shift rotation is difficult for shift workers because just as the biological clock starts adjusting to one shift, it must then completely resynchronize to a new shift (see Chapter 2). Weekly circadian changes keep the biological clock in a permanent state of flux and unable to reach its goal of optimal circadian adjustment. If the weekly rotation follows phase advances (nights-to-evenings-to-days), the shift schedule may pose even greater difficulties for the biological clock.

Choosing a Shift System

From all of the available evidence, we know that weekly rotation should be avoided even when only two shifts are involved, as is most common in nursing organizations. The choices left to nurse administrators, then, are fixed shifts, slowly rotating shifts, or rapidly rotating shifts. In general, performance studies of night shift nurses support voluntary fixed shifts (see Chapter 6). The nurse's ability to select a shift and his or her level of commitment to shift work (based on social, professional, domestic, educational, or financial reasons) are two important factors in recommending a voluntary permanent shift system. In many cases, nurses who cannot adapt to fixed night shifts will request an in-house transfer or resign; for a variety of reasons, not all do this. Because some nurses who cannot adapt to night work still attempt to remain on fixed night shifts, nurse managers have an obligation to monitor the performance of night shift nurses in order to ensure that patient safety and productivity standards are maintained. Nurse administrators also have an obligation to encourage the use of self-selection and education (including information on the coping strategies described in Chapter 8) to increase the likelihood that volunteers for permanent night shifts will succeed in their positions.

Although we know that some nurse administrators make involuntary nursing assignments to fixed night shifts, the consequences of this practice have not been adequately studied. Until nurse researchers can provide more information about the effects of involuntary permanent night shift work on nurses' performance and retention, we recommend that either slowly or rapidly rotating shift workers be used to supplement the voluntary permanent night shift staff.

While both slow and rapid shift rotation systems have advantages and disadvantages, each can be modified to meet the needs of a particular nursing staff and nursing unit. Since both systems are used by millions of shift workers worldwide, neither should be rejected solely on the basis of personal prejudice. We know that peak performance of more complex tasks occurs earlier in the day for diurnally-oriented individuals, and that performance involving memory tasks and verbal and mathematical reasoning adjusts to time shifts more quickly than performance involving simple repetitive or vigilance tasks. Therefore, rapid rotation should be considered for nurses who perform highly cognitive tasks, such as therapeutic decision making and drug dosage calculations in critical care units. Rotating 12-hour shifts usually resemble the rapid rotation pattern if a nurse reverts to nighttime sleep on days off. Slow rotations are generally preferred for monitoring, inspection, and quality control tasks (Monk, 1986). Although slow rotation has physiological adaptation advantages when compared to more rapidly rotating shift systems, social and domestic problems often arise with longer rotations to night shift work, particularly for nurses with children at home.

In order to choose the most effective shift system, nurse administrators also must consider the advantages of self-scheduling and unit-designed schedules that are based on group preferences. Schedules designed by unit staff were found to be more successful in preventing turnover than permanent shifts or computer-generated schedules that were based on staffing requests and preset daily unit needs (Choi et al., 1986). Nurse researchers need to evaluate the differences between schedules based on circadian rhythms theory and computer-generated schedules based on nurses' preferences and unit needs (Kostreva and Genevier, 1989).

Shift Selection Factors

While we cannot definitely predict who will adapt well to shift work and who will not, we do know quite a bit about the social and health risk factors associated with shift work coping problems. Chapters 4 and 7 reviewed the existing health disorders and the individual characteristics and social factors identified by Scott and LaDou (1990) as definite or relative contraindications for shift work. This information can be used for many beneficial purposes:

- by prospective shift workers to assess the probability of their success in coping with night work;
- by nurse administrators to counsel nurse applicants about fixed and rotating night shift positions;
- by staff educators to prepare orientation and shift work adaptation programs; and
- by nurse researchers to continue investigating the predictive ability of these risk factors to differentiate between who will and will not adapt to shift work.

We know several nurses with one or more of the contraindications for shift work who have managed to successfully adjust to night work; therefore, Scott and LaDou's lists of contraindications should not be used to summarily exclude nurses from working particular shifts. However, because the consequences of poor adjustment to night work may be more serious for those nurses with some existing medical conditions, we recommend obtaining medical clearance from the nurse's private physician or the employee health service before assigning these individuals to permanent or rotating night shifts. Rotation to evening shifts may be preferable in order to optimize the health of these nurses. Employee health service staff should be sensitive to shift work problems and their treatment, as well as cognizant of the symptoms of drug abuse, alcoholism, and family stress that may be associated with poor adjustment to shift work.

As discussed in Chapter 7, the amount of sleep each individual needs is another shift selection factor. Nurse recruiters and managers should be aware of individual sleep requirements when counseling prospective night or rotating shift nurses. Nurses requiring more than eight or nine hours of sleep a day should be encouraged to work evening rather than night shifts. Because patient safety is threatened when nurses are sleep-deprived, nurse administrators should discourage secondary positions for full-time night shift nurses, and should avoid asking such nurses to work double shifts, particularly between two consecutive night shifts.

In Chapter 7, we also recommended that nurses' shift work assessments include measuring their chronotype through the Circadian Type Questionnaire. Nurse administrators should encourage the use of the CTQ and its scoring sheet for those interested in evaluating their circadian type (see Figure 7.3).

Staff Education

Although most of this chapter concerns evaluating and choosing shift systems, it is vital for nurse administrators to realize that their responsibility to nurse shift workers does not end there. The intent of this book is to underscore the fact that shift work self-assessment, the development and implementation of shift work coping strategies, staff education, and an open approach to communication are equally important and can all benefit shift workers, nurse administrators and, ultimately, patients. The director of nursing staff development can be the chief proponent for this approach to shift work by developing a Nurses' Shift Work Adaptation Program for the organization (see Chapter 8). The NSWAP should be thoroughly discussed with and understood by all nursing staff assigned to shift work, whether on a fixed or rotating basis.

Any in-service programs that are offered during the day should also be offered during the night at times convenient for the evening and night shift nursing staff. Based on the research findings reviewed in Chapter 2, educational classes should be held early in the night shift (not at 4:00 a.m.) to be of the most benefit to nurse shift workers. Night shift nurses have frequently told us that they are overlooked when in-service classes are scheduled, and that their needs and interests are not considered when program content is developed. Videotapes and self-study modules can make it possible to tailor classes to the needs and work schedules of individual shift workers.

Support for Nurse Shift Workers

Steps should be taken to ensure that shift workers do not feel that they are treated as "second-class citizens." Nurse administrators need to make sure that nurse shift workers are not denied access to staff or committee meetings, professional education classes, employee health clinics, cafeteria services, or recreational activities simply by virtue of their shift schedules. In general, the night shift nurses we interviewed for this book believe that they are an essential part of the provision of quality patient care; however, they feel somewhat isolated from and overlooked by nurse executives, educators, and researchers. Permanent night shift nurses would welcome more participation in nursing committee work, quality improvement programs, and clinical research activities; scheduling some nursing activities early in the day or late in the afternoon would facilitate their participation in activities that cannot be scheduled during the night.

If day shift employees have access to smoking cessation, weight control, physical fitness, or other wellness clinics, these opportunities should also be made accessible to and convenient for evening and night shift workers. The morale of shift workers often can be enormously boosted simply by providing vending machines with nutritious food choices and microwave ovens to heat the food. An even better alternative is to keep the cafeteria open for most of the night in order to provide hot meals for night shift workers. More large hospitals should consider the feasibility of meeting this need. Additionally, based on preliminary studies of bright light treatment (see Chapter 8), the areas where night shift nurses work, eat meals, and take breaks should have increased illumination levels.

Counseling services and self-help groups should be accessible to night shift workers. Questionnaires can be developed to help night shift nurses with medical, psychological, and social self-surveillance. Scott and LaDou (1990) recommend yearly surveillance for most shift workers, with an emphasis on identifying symptoms of sleep deprivation, domestic and social conflicts, and medical disorders incompatible with night work (see Chapter 4).

Summary

Nurse administrators need to be sophisticated in their approach to the shift system in their particular health care facility. They should choose shift systems that are appropriate and beneficial to their nursing personnel, and should work with employee health and safety personnel, staff educators, and nurse researchers to develop educational and counseling mechanisms for ensuring the health, safety, and job satisfaction of nurse shift workers. An important goal is to prevent isolating evening and night shift nurses from their day shift colleagues. Finally, nurse administrators should realize that enhancing the personal and professional well-being of nurse shift workers is a cost-effective contribution to quality patient care.

— Chapter 10 —

Shift Work Policies

Introduction

N urses, their health care colleagues, and patients who are
engaged in shift work in the United States and Canada
have very little protection through existing laws, regulations, or policies related to shift work. There are no general working
condition standards for shift workers in North America; however,
there is some federal work schedule protection in certain U.S. industries (e.g., the transportation and nuclear power industries) where
public safety is an important concern, and there are some provincial
regulations in Canada. This type of work schedule protection has
not been extended to health care workers in either country, although the actions of these workers, when sleep-deprived, can also
threaten the public safety. Most of the protection from shift work
hazards that is afforded to registered nurses in North America
comes from local collective bargaining agreements and from enlight-
ened nurse management policies. In this chapter, we will discuss
shift work policies from international, national, nurses' association,
and nursing management perspectives.

International Shift Work Policies

For over 100 years, there have been international attempts to
regulate working conditions, particularly for women and children.

In 1890, a resolution prohibiting night work by women was passed by the International Congress for the Protection of Workers. In 1919, the International Labor Organization (ILO) was established and passed its first convention (international treaty) limiting working hours for both men and women to 48 hours per week and eight hours per day. Since that time, the ILO has adopted three additional conventions regulating night work by women (U.S. Congress, 1991).

Although previous conventions were concerned with night work in specific industries and working conditions for women and young people in particular, the first ILO regulations on general night work for all workers were adopted in 1990. Several of the requirements of this 1990 convention are of interest to night shift nurses in light of similar recommendations made in this book. The convention requirements included medical surveillance before and during night work assignments, and accessible social and counseling services to facilitate adaptation to night work, especially with regard to sleeping, meals, and off-duty activities. Nonbinding propositions included limiting night work to eight hours in a 24-hour period, guaranteeing at least 11 hours between shifts, avoiding overtime and double shifts for night workers, providing facilities for meals and rest, minimizing commuting time, and arranging for educational leave and training (U.S. Congress, 1991).

The 1990 ILO convention also adopted a revision of an earlier prohibition against industrial night work by women, with exemptions for emergency work, managerial jobs, technical tasks, and nonmanual health occupations. Thus, the nursing profession is allowed to work at night in countries that ratified this convention. The 1990 revision allows the earlier restrictions on night work by women to be superseded by collective bargaining agreements and legislation, although it prohibits night work for at least eight weeks before childbirth, and for a total of 16 weeks before and after childbirth. This is considerably less restrictive than the 1978 ILO Tripartite Advisory Meeting on Night Work, which made a unanimous call for prohibiting night work entirely by pregnant women.

The ILO, now an agency of the United Nations, not only formulates conventions and recommendations, but also assists its 152 member nations in implementing labor standards through technical assistance, training, and special programs. If a country ratifies an ILO convention, it is required to implement the regulations and report related activities to the ILO. Alternatively, member nations can denounce a convention or merely ignore it. Many countries' protective labor regulations for women, children, and workers in general are modeled on ILO conventions (U.S. Congress, 1991).

National Shift Work Policies

Nations that regulate shift work do so through four basic methods and combinations thereof:

1) national legislation,
2) national collective bargaining agreements through a single union representing all workers,
3) regional or local legislation, and /or
4) local collective bargaining agreements.

Countries show great variation in the degree and substance of their shift work laws, regulations, and policies. The continuum ranges from nations with extensive regulations covering even shift workers' housing, leisure facilities, and retirement programs, to countries with little or no national regulations (U.S. Congress, 1991).

National legislation mandating increased pay and fewer hours for nonstandard work schedules are the most common form of shift work regulation. For example, Korean law requires a 50% pay differential for night work, and Finland and Sweden require night shifts to be two hours shorter than day shifts (U.S. Congress, 1991). Many nations have more laws regulating night and shift work for women and young people than for men.

Several European countries have extensive general shift work regulations. Austrian law requires 11 uninterrupted hours of rest between shifts, and night workers receive extra shift breaks, two to six extra vacation days a year, and a special pension. Additionally, every Austrian company employing more than 50 shift workers in heavy manual labor must have an on-site medical officer. France has laws mandating a medical examination before shift work is undertaken, and requiring special food arrangements for shift workers. French night workers are subsidized for making their homes soundproof and lightproof, and some French television programs are rebroadcast for night shift workers. France also requires that night workers be given priority for national housing funds (U.S. Congress, 1991). In Japan, certain night workers are legally allowed to sleep on company time. West Germany has one of the most rigid set of regulations in the word regarding airline pilot duty hours. Also in West Germany, large industrial plants offer middle-aged shift workers two- to three-week stays at special treatment centers, where these workers are able to normalize their biological clocks and receive physiotherapy and health examinations at company expense.

In other European countries, shift work is illegal for women, although there are often exceptions for health care and other special workers. Employers must obtain a permit to hire female shift workers, and the granting of that permit can be made conditional on the employer providing adequate conditions, benefits, and services for shift workers. When discrimination against women was barred by civil rights legislation in the 1970s, European experts seriously considered whether equality should be attained by including men in the shift work ban, rather than by abolishing the ban for women (Monk, 1988).

Not all of the regulations that countries impose on shift workers are desirable from a perspective of chronobiological well-being. Switzerland, for example, limits consecutive night shifts to six weeks, and Iraq has a one-month limit on consecutive night shifts, thereby effectively banning permanent night shift work. Several countries' regulations encourage weekly shift rotations. At present, no nation requires that shift rotation be in the more desirable direction of days-to-evenings-to-nights, and none demands extra time off at the end of a night rotation (U.S. Congress, 1991).

The United States and Canada are two of the nations that have not ratified the ILO convention regulating shift work for women. Neither country has national regulations for general shift work, although there is some federal protective legislation in the United States for workers in the railroad, trucking, commercial airline, air traffic control, and nuclear power industries. In both countries, many regulations governing working conditions are under the jurisdiction of states and provinces rather than the federal government. The U.S. Equal Employment Opportunity Commission determined that state laws prohibiting night work by women violated Title VII of the Civil Rights Act of 1969, which forbids discrimination based on sex, race, or religion. Thus, the 20 states that had laws restricting night work by women repealed them in the 1970s (U.S. Congress, 1991).

Nurses Association Policies

The American Nurses Association, as a federation of state nurses associations, has no national standards or guidelines on shift work, although consultation on workplace advocacy issues is offered to state nurses associations and their members. In many instances, the only regulation of shift work policies for registered nurses in this country occurs through participation in local collective bargaining agreements. The American Hospital Association (1992) reports that in 1990, approximately 17% of short-term, acute care hospitals in the United States recognized collective bargaining for their RN staffs. Almost half of these bargaining units were represented by state nurses associations.

The amount and type of work schedule protection included in local collective bargaining agreements negotiated by nurses in America show considerable variation. Each unit bargains over choice of shifts, shift assignments, time between shifts, split shifts, and shift rotations (U.S. Congress, 1991). Commonly included in the "hours of work" section of a nursing contract are limits on the number of different shifts worked in a week, limits on shift rotation for seniority, and the required number of hours between shifts. The "compensation" section of such contracts generally contains provisions for shift differential payments. Without national or state legislation regulating shift work, however, collective bargaining units are not always successful in obtaining major shift work guarantees for their nurse members.

Nursing Management Policies

There is very little published information concerning current U.S. nursing management policies on shift work. From the many interviews we conducted for this book, however, we know that the continuum of management policies extends from an "anything goes" lack of policy, to policies requiring all permanent or rotating shift assignments for most of the nursing staff. Some nursing organizations have centralized policies regarding shift rotation; many others are decentralized to the nursing unit level. About one-third of all registered nurses working in short-term, acute care hospitals in 1990 worked some type of rotating shift (American Hospital Association, 1992), an insignificant change from 1988 numbers (Adams, 1989). What did noticeably change between 1988 and 1990 was the percentage of hospital nurses rotating to all three shifts — this percentage decreased from 14.5% in 1988 to 10.7% in 1990 (see Table 10.1).

A qualitative study of the shift work practices of 23 nurse executives from urban and rural U.S. hospitals found that most had policies requiring shift rotation, generally between either days and evenings or days and nights. Only one nurse administrator in this sample expected RNs to rotate to all three shifts. Platoon-like, routinized patterns were not used in these nursing organizations, and some had self-scheduling policies in place. The majority of the nurse administrators in this study expected nurses to rotate shifts within a week, and only a few used slow rotation patterns. Days off varied during the week, but the majority of nurses had every other weekend off. The reason most commonly given by this sample of nurse administrators for rapid and weekly rotations, flexible patterning, and self-scheduling was that nurses with families found long periods of night shift rotation to be a burden. Schedule flexibility was most valued by nurses who were responsible for child care and by those nurses who were part-time students. Only a small percentage of the nurse administrators in this study ever assigned nurses to permanent shifts. In comparison to the shift work practices of the other four industries researched, the investigators of this study gave hospital nurse administrators credit for being more innovative and flexible (McLaughlin and Mohr, 1988).

In some cases, shift rotation continues because nurse administrators believe that this policy is best for patient care and the harmony of the nursing staff. It was the opinion of one administrator we interviewed that after 5–10 years of permanent night shift work, negative interpersonal relationships can develop between nurses on different shifts. To avoid an "us/them" relationship between groups of shift workers, this particular nurse administrator preferred for nurses to rotate to other shifts occasionally. Another nurse administrator we interviewed stated that patients deserved the same standard of care at night as they received during the day, and that the best way to ensure this was to avoid permanent night shift assignments by rotating all nurses.

After interviewing over 80 night shift nurses and nurse administrators for this book, we perceive a slight trend toward less shift rotation in nursing organizations. To encourage nurses to accept permanent night work, or at least very slow rotations, many nurse administrators have instituted special compensation packages, which can include bonus payments, extra paid days off on a weekly or monthly basis, and higher pay differentials for working at least three months of night shifts. If a nurse administrator determines that permanent shift assignments are possible according to the number of RNs requesting or agreeing to work fixed evening or night shifts (or a 12-hour night shift in some cases), a policy of "no rotations except in emergencies" may be adopted. The advantages of such a policy include less sleep deprivation, increased job satisfaction, and improved retention. Many nurses request permanent night shift work to accommodate their child care or education schedules, and prefer it to rotating shift assignments. Other nurses, particularly those who are single or married without children, told us that they would rather rotate between days and one other shift than be involuntarily assigned to a fixed night or evening shift. Vacancies in fixed evening and night shifts accounted for 53.1% of all hospital nurse vacancies in 1990 (American Hospital Association, 1992).

Because most of the shift work regulation that is in effect for North American RNs occurs through collective bargaining agreements, we should also mention the nurse administrator's role in contract negotiation. While registered nurses seek flexible schedules and major guarantees, nursing management also tries to preserve flexibility in staffing nursing units. Therefore, all nurses understand that a complete elimination of shift rotation is difficult to negotiate. The general trend in management policies seems to be toward decentralized structures and self-scheduling, rather than toward rigid policies that either require or prohibit shift rotation.

A Call for Political Action

Despite the approximately 20 million U.S. voters who work non-standard schedules (U.S. Congress, 1991), there has been very little activity on Capitol Hill regarding shift work. In Chapter 6, we mentioned a Congressional subcommittee hearing on shift work, the proceedings of which were published and then largely ignored. Much of that 1983 testimony would sound familiar to readers of this book: shift workers told of fatigue, family problems, and digestive ailments; regulators and association representatives questioned the safety of patient care, air transportation, and nuclear power stations; and all spoke of the need for more shift work information for employers, workers, and regulators. The second Congressional action of any significance regarding shift work was the 1991 report by the Office of Technology Assessment on the implications of biological rhythms for workers (U.S. Congress, 1991). Registered nurses were the subject of one of the case studies in this report.

Because the majority of shift work studies have not included North American nurses as subjects, funding is needed so that the National Institute for Nursing Research, the Division of Nursing, or the Department of Labor can sponsor specific investigations of nurse shift workers. One of the areas that needs to be researched more thoroughly involves the amount of shift work policy flexibility that should be retained by employers and shift workers, and the areas of shift work that should be regulated. Other important topics for research include whether shift work has different adverse effects on men and women, and whether there should be either general or specific protective regulations for shift workers.

Individual nurses should inform their federal and state legislators that the United States lags behind the rest of the industrialized world in shift work legislation and regulations that protect the worker (U.S. Congress, 1991). [This is also true of Canada.] Reminding legislators that shift workers represent a sizable portion of their constituencies may help raise some interest in this topic.

Summary

The success of attempts to establish international shift work standards has been limited by the reluctance of some nations to be bound by regulations. The United States and Canada, for instance, have far fewer shift work regulations and policies than many other industrialized countries. In the few U.S. industries with shift work regulations, the United States is the leader in the trend toward legislation that protects men and women equally (Singer, 1989). This legislation either extends shift work protection to men or removes it from women.

Much of the shift work regulation for RNs in the United States occurs through local collective bargaining agreements, although the majority of U.S. registered nurses are dependent on the shift work policies of nursing management to protect them from the hazards of shift work. We hope that the content of this book will serve to enlighten both registered nurses and nurse administrators as they work together to create policies that protect nurse shift workers and the patients they care for around the clock.

FIGURE 10.1

Percentages of Registered Nurses Working Fixed and Rotating Shifts in U.S. Hospitals

	1988	**1990**
Fixed Day Shift	28.9%	31.2%
Fixed Evening Shift	20.8%	18.3%
Fixed Night Shift	17.4%	18.0%
Total, Fixed Shifts	67.1%	67.5%
Rotate to Days and Evenings	8.8%	10.9%
Rotate to Days and Nights	6.9%	7.1%
Rotate to Evenings and Nights	2.7%	3.9%
Rotate to Days, Evenings, and Nights	14.5%	10.7%
Total, Rotating Shifts	32.9%	32.6%

Sources: 1) C. Adams, 1989, *Report of the Hospital Nursing Personnel Surveys*, Chicago: American Hospital Association; and 2) American Hospital Association, 1992, *1990 Report of the Hospital Nursing Personnel Survey*, Chicago: American Hospital Association.

Epilogue

W hen we first began work on this book several years ago, we were acutely aware of how little information was available to those nurses eager to learn how to better cope with shift work. This awareness was reinforced by our personal experiences conducting studies of shift-working nurses in England, New York, and Virginia. Recent interviews with over 80 shift-working nurses around the country convinced us that nursing shift work problems are widespread and real, and that the need for information and solutions is overwhelming.

So much of the literature on shift work is found in obscure journals and periodicals, in which the central findings are made complex by technical jargon and unusual chronobiological terms and concepts. Through this book, we hope to have engaged the intellectual curiosity of nurses without drowning them in a sea of complicated and irrelevant details. We have tried to neither overcomplicate nor oversimplify shift work problems and strategies. Though it is always more convenient to receive a ready-made solution, we have attempted to guide the reader toward a personalized solution to shift work problems, through:

- understanding the background material related to shift work,
- evaluating shift work problems and his or her personal relationship to them, and
- developing coping strategies for all of the various shift work problem areas.

We firmly believe that this hands-on approach is necessary for a topic as multifaceted as shift work, and that members of the nursing profession are both willing and able to benefit from it.

We conclude this book by wishing you much success in developing your own NSWAP — swapping an old life-style and shift work approach for a new and more productive outlook. We hope that your NSWAP will bring you significant and long-lasting gains in health, well-being, and satisfaction at work and home. Good luck!

Glossary*

Adaptation. The process of adjusting an individual's biological clock to a timing appropriate to that individual's daily routine. See *Phase Shift*.

Afternoon Shift. See *Evening Shift*.

Amplitude of Rhythm. As it relates to circadian rhythms, the difference between the maximum or minimum and mean values of a function (e.g., body temperature) during the circadian cycle. Amplitude provides a measure of extent of the fluctuation within a cycle. See *Circadian Rhythm*.

Apnea. A sleep disorder that involves the repeated cessation of breathing during the night (often associated with loud snoring). Each episode causes a transient arousal from sleep that can leave the patient excessively sleepy during the day.

Arousal Model. A model which postulates that circadian rhythms in performance efficiency during the day are mediated via changes in basal arousal that are broadly parallel to changes in body temperature.

Backward Rotation. Changes in shifts from nights to evenings to days. Compare *Forward Rotation*.

---

*This glossary draws heavily from previous glossaries by Monk and Folkard (1992) and U.S. Congress (1991).

Biological Clock. The internal mechanism of the body that controls biological rhythms. See *Circadian Pacemaker.*

Biological Rhythm. A self-sustained, cyclical change in a physiological process or behavioral function that repeats at regular intervals. See *Circadian Rhythm, Infradian Rhythm, Ultradian Rhythm.*

Biorhythm Theory. A theory that postulates three infradian rhythms that control human behavior and performance. It has no scientific basis.

Bright Light. Bright light has been shown to shift circadian rhythms and has been used to treat some sleep disorders and jet lag. In order to affect human circadian rhythms in a strong way, the bright light needs to have an intensity of at least 2,500 lux, which is equivalent to outdoor light at dawn.

Chronobiologist. One who studies *Chronobiology.*

Chronobiology. The scientific study of the effect of time on living systems, including the study of biological rhythms.

Chronopharmacologist. A chronobiologist who specializes in the study of circadian rhythms in medication efficacy and toxicity.

Chronopsychologist. A chronobiologist who specializes in the study of circadian rhythms in mood, activation, and performance.

Chronotype. A classification of individuals as either *Morning Larks* or *Night Owls.* Also referred to as *Circadian Type.*

Circadian. Having a period of about one day (from the Latin: circa dies). See *Circadian Pacemaker, Circadian Rhythm.*

Circadian Pacemaker. The part of the brain responsible for the generation of circadian signals. See *Circadian Rhythm, Suprachiasmatic Nucleus.*

Circadian Rhythm. A self-sustained biological rhythm which, in a natural environment, is normally synchronized to a 24-hour period. See *Biological Rhythm.*

Circadian Type. A classification of individuals as either *Morning Larks* or *Night Owls.* Also referred to as *Chronotype.*

Comparatively Rapid Rotation. A rotating shift schedule that involves three or four consecutive shifts at one timing before moving to a different timing.

Constant Conditions Protocol. An experiment in which an individual is kept awake but in bed for 36–48 hours without knowledge of clock time. This allows a more accurate measurement of *Endogenous Circadian Rhythms.*

Continental Rotation. See *Rapid Rotation.*

Cortisol. A steroid hormone secreted by humans. Cortisol secretion exhibits a circadian rhythm and is used as a marker for the body's pacemaker.

Cyclical Rotation Patterns. Workday and shift assignments that are predictable and repetitious.

Day Shift. A period of work in which half or more of the hours worked occur between 8:00 a.m. and 4:00 p.m.

Delta Sleep. See *Slow Wave Sleep.*

Diurnal. Active during the day.

Double Jobbing. See *Moonlighting, Secondary Position.*

Double Shift. Two consecutive shifts worked in a single 24-hour period.

EEG. Electroencephalogram. The pattern of changes in electrical potential as measured by electrodes placed on the scalp.

EMG. Electromyogram. The pattern of changes in electrical potential as measured by electrodes placed on the skin near muscles (chin muscles in the case of sleep recording).

Endogenous Circadian Rhythm. Circadian Rhythms that are the result of internal physiological processes rather than responses to changes in waking state, posture, or activity.

EOG. Electrooculogram. The pattern of changes in electrical potential generated by eye movements, as detected by electrodes placed near the eyes. Used to detect *Rapid Eye Movement (REM) Sleep.*

Epoch. A unit of time used to divide a sleep record. Typical epochs are of a 30–60 second duration. Each epoch is scored into a particular sleep stage.

Evening Person. A general term used to describe an individual who has difficulty waking up in the morning, is able to sleep late, and finds it difficult to fall asleep at night. Also referred to as *Night Owl.* Compare *Morning Lark.*

Evening Shift. A period of work, more than half of which occurs after 4:00 p.m.

Fatigue. Weariness caused by physical and mental exertion.

Fixed Shift. A work schedule in which the hours of work remain the same from day to day. Also referred to as *Permanent Shift*. Compare *Irregular Shift, Rotating Shift*.

Forward Rotation. Changes in shifts from days to evenings to nights. Compare *Backward Rotation*.

Free-Running. A circadian rhythm operating in the absence of environmental cues. Such rhythms may last 20–28 hours. Under free-running conditions, the human body clock has a circadian rhythm of about 25 hours, although this varies with age, gender, and circadian type.

Homeostasis. The view that the internal physiological environment is utterly constant. The presence of circadian rhythms reveals that this view needs revision.

Individual Differences. Differences between one person and another because of age, gender, personality, circadian type, or other attribute.

Infradian Rhythm. A biological rhythm with a cycle of more than 24 hours (the menstrual cycle, for example). See *Biological Rhythm;* compare *Ultradian Rhythm*.

Internal Dissociation. The loss of harmony between the component parts of the circadian system, leading to symptoms like those of *Jet Lag*.

Irregular Shift. A work schedule that is variable and unpredictable. Compare *Fixed Shift, Rotating Shift*.

Jet Lag. The malaise associated with travel across time zones. It results from conflict between the traveler's internal clock and the external rhythms in the new time zone.

Melatonin. A hormone produced by the pineal gland, which is present in many animals, including humans. Melatonin secretion is circadian, and production is readily inhibited by bright light. Melatonin is being investigated as a possible circadian entraining agent in humans. See *Zeitgeber*.

Metropolitan Rotation. See *Rapid Rotation*.

Moonlighting. Holding more than one paid job at the same time.

132

Morning Lark. A general term used to describe an individual who wakes up easily, has difficulty sleeping late, and falls asleep quickly at night. Compare *Evening Person.*

Multi-Oscillator. Having more than one controlling oscillator. In circadian terms, having more than one *Circadian Pacemaker.*

Night Shift Paralysis. A rare condition marked by short-term paralysis, usually lasting about two minutes, during which individuals are aware of their surroundings but are unable to move. This condition is associated with extreme sleep deprivation.

Night Owl. See *Evening Person.*

Night Shift. A period of work in which half or more of the hours worked occur between midnight and 8:00 a.m.

Nocturnal. Active at night.

Nocturnal Myoclonus. Periodic sudden jerks and involuntary movements of the legs during the night, which can lead to disrupted sleep.

NSWAP. Nurses' Shift Work Awareness Program. An educational program designed to promote awareness of shift work issues and coping techniques.

Peak of Rhythm. The highest value of a rhythmic variable.

Period. The length of time that elapses before a rhythm repeats itself.

Permanent Shift. See *Fixed Shift.*

Phase Adjustment. See *Phase Shift.*

Phase Advance. Movement of a rhythm to an earlier timing of peak and trough. See *Phase Shift.*

Phase Delay. Movement of a rhythm to a later timing of peak and trough. See *Phase Shift.*

Phase Shift. The resetting of an individual's internal clock in response to an entraining agent. Circadian rhythms may be advanced, delayed, or not shifted at all, depending on the timing of exposure. See *Phase Advance, Phase Delay, Zeitgeber,*

Pineal Gland. A small structure in the brain that produces the hormone melatonin. In some species, such as birds, it is the *Circadian Pacemaker.*

Polysomnographic Measures. Measures taken during sleep by amplifying EEG, EMG, and EOG signals from electrodes placed on the head, and plotting the resultant waves out on a polygraph. These measures are used to score sleep into stages.

Rapid Eye Movement (REM) Sleep. Stage of sleep during which the eyes move rapidly and brain activity resembles that observed during wakefulness. Heart rate and respiration increase and become erratic, and vivid dreams are frequent. REM sleep alternates with non-REM sleep in ultradian cycles lasting from 90–100 minutes. Compare *Slow Wave Sleep.*

Rapid Rotation. A rotating shift schedule that involves only one or two shifts at one timing before moving to a different timing. Compare *Fixed Shift.*

REM Sleep. See *Rapid Eye Movement Sleep.*

REM Rebound. An increase in *Rapid Eye Movement (REM) Sleep* on a night following a period of REM suppression.

Rotating Shifts. A shift schedule in which the hours of work change regularly; for example, from day to evening to night shifts. Rotation may be rapid (e.g., every three days), medium (e.g., every week), or slow (e.g., every four weeks), and may be forward or backward. See *Forward Rotation, Backward Rotation;* compare *Fixed Shift, Irregular Shift.*

Secondary Position. See *Double Jobbing, Moonlighting.*

Shift Maladaptation Syndrome (SMS). A combination of ailments arising from the inability of some workers to adjust to long-term shift work.

Shift System. The way in which work schedules are organized in order to provide the desired coverage.

Shift Work. Used in this book to refer to any nonstandard work schedule (including evening or night shifts, rotating shifts, split shifts, and extended duty hours) in which the hours of work commonly or always occur outside the period between 7:00 a.m. and 6:00 p.m.

Sleep Apnea. See *Apnea.*

Sleep Deprivation. Lack of sufficient sleep.

Sleep Rigidity/Flexibility. An individual's ability to vary the timing of his or her sleep episode.

Sleep Stages. The way in which various types and depths of sleep are categorized using *Polysomnographic Measures.*

Slow Rotation. A rotating shift schedule that involves two or more consecutive weeks on one shift timing before moving to a different shift timing.

Slow Wave Sleep. The stages of sleep during which slow delta waves appear on the EEG, the eyes do not move, heart rate and respiration are slow and steady, muscles show little movement, and dreams are infrequent. Compare *Rapid Eye Movement (REM) Sleep.*

Spontaneous Internal Desynchronization. A phenomenon observed in *Free-Running*, time-isolated individuals whose circadian temperature rhythms run at a radically different period length than that of their sleep-wake cycle.

Strain. See *Stressor.*

Stressor. Any source of stress. Used in this book primarily to refer to the disruption of circadian rhythms, the disruption of sleep, and the social and domestic disturbances caused by shift work.

Suprachiasmatic Nucleus. The region of a mammal's brain that acts as the primary circadian pacemaker, controlling or coordinating circadian rhythms. See *Circadian Pacemaker.*

Transmeridian Flight. Travel across time zones. See *Jet Lag.*

Trough of Rhythm. The lowest value of a rhythmic variable.

Ultradian Rhythm. A biological rhythm with a cycle of less than 24 hours. Human sleep cycles and the release of some hormones are examples.

Variable Schedule. A shift schedule in which the timing of the shift follows no predictable pattern.

Vigilance. The task of maintaining alert watchfulness in an inherently routine and/or sleep-inducing situation.

Weekly Rotation. A rotating shift schedule that involves between five and seven consecutive shifts at one timing before moving to a different shift timing.

Zeitgeber. A factor that synchronizes an organism's biological rhythms to the outside world; for example, the light-dark cycle is an entraining agent for circadian rhythms.

References

Adams, C. 1989. *Report of the Hospital Nursing Personnel Surveys: 1988 summary of major findings.* Chicago: American Hospital Association.

Adams, J.; Folkard, S.; and Young, M. 1986. Coping strategies used by nurses on night duty. *Ergonomics* 29:185-196.

Akerstedt, T. 1985. Adjustment of physiological circadian rhythms and the sleep-wake cycle to shiftwork. In *Hours of work: Temporal factors in work scheduling,* eds. S. Folkard and T.H. Monk, pp. 185-197. New York: John Wiley & Sons.

Akerstedt, T. and Gillberg, M. 1981. The circadian variation of experimentally displaced sleep. *Sleep* 4:159-169.

Alward, R.R. 1986. Performance of permanent versus rotating night nurses: Circadian-related factors. Doctoral dissertation, Teachers College, Columbia University, New York, N.Y.

_____.1988. Are you a lark or an owl on the night shift? *American Journal of Nursing* 88:1336-1339.

Alward, R.R. and Monk, T.H. 1990. A comparison of rotating-shift and permanent night nurses. *International Journal of Nursing Studies* 27:297-302.

American Hospital Association. 1992. *1990 report of the Hospital Nursing Personnel Survey.* Chicago: American Hospital Association.

Anch, A.M.; Browman, C.P.; Mitler, M.M.; and Walsh, J.K. 1988. *Sleep: A scientific perspective.* Englewood Cliffs, N.J.: Prentice-Hall.

Arendt, J.; Minors, D.S.; and Waterhouse, J.M. 1989. Basic concepts and implications. In *Biological rhythms in clinical practice,* eds. J. Arendt, D.S. Minors, and J.M. Waterhouse, pp. 3-7.London: Wright.

Aschoff, J.; Hoffman, K.; Pohl, H.; and Wever, R.A. 1975. Re-entrainment of circadian rhythms after phase-shifts of the zeitgeber. *Chronobiologia* 2:23-78.

Aserinsky, E. and Kleitman, N. 1953. Regularly occuring periods of eye motility and concomitant phenomena during sleep. *Science* 118:273.

Baddeley, A.D. 1968. A three-minute reasoning test based on grammatical transformation. *Psychonomic Science* 10:341.

Baddeley, A.D.; Hatter, J.E.; Scott, D.; and Snashall, A. 1970. Memory and time of day. *Quarterly Journal of Experimental Psychology* 22:605-609.

Bjerner, B. and Swensson, A. 1953. Shiftwork and rhythm. *Acta Medica Scandinavica* 278:102-107.

Blake, M.J.F. 1967. Time of day effects on performance in a range of tasks. *Psychonomic Science* 9:349-350.

Borbély, A.A. 1982. A two-process model of sleep regulation. *Human Neurobiology* 1:195-204.

Bosch, L.H.M. and de Lange, W.A.M. 1987. Shift work in health care. *Ergonomics* 30:773-791.

Broughton, R.J. 1989. Chronobiological aspects and models of sleep and napping. In *Sleep and alertness: Chronobiological, behavioral, and medical aspects of napping,* eds. D.F. Dinges and Broughton, R.J., pp. 71-98. New York: Raven Press.

Browne, R.C. 1949. The day and night performance of tele-printer switchboard operators. *Occupational Psychology* 23:121-126.

Buysse, D.J. 1991. Drugs affecting sleep, sleepiness and performance. In *Sleep, sleepiness and performance,* ed. T.H. Monk, pp. 249-306. Chichester, England: John Wiley & Sons.

Campbell, S.S. 1984. Duration and placement of sleep in a "disentrained" environment. *Psychophysiology* 21:106-113.

Carskadon, M.A. and Dement, W.C. 1992. Multiple sleep latency tests during the constant routine. *Sleep* 15(6):396-399.

Carskadon, M.A. and Roth, T. 1991. Sleep restriction. In *Sleep, sleepiness and performance,* ed. T.H. Monk, pp. 155-167. Chichester, England: John Wiley & Sons.

Choi, T.; Jameson, H.; Brekke, M.; Podratz, R.; and Mundahl, H. 1986. Effects on nurse retention: An experiment with scheduling. *Medical Care* 24:1029-1043.

Coffey, L.C.; Skipper, J.K.; and Jung, F.D. 1988. Nurses and shift work: Effects on job performance and job-related stress. *Journal of Advanced Nursing* 13:245-254.

Cole, R.J.; Loving, R.T.; and Kripke, D.F. 1990. Psychiatric aspects of shiftwork. *Occupational Medicine* 5:301-314.

Colligan, M.J. and Rosa, R.R. 1990. Shiftwork effects on social and family life. *Occupational Medicine* 5:315-322.

Colquhoun, W.P. 1971. Circadian variations in mental efficiency. In *Biological rhythms and human performance,* ed. W.P. Colquhoun, pp. 39-107. London: Academic Press.

Conroy, R.T.W.L. and Mills, J.N. 1970. *Human circadian rhythms.* London: Churchill.

Czeisler, C.A.; Brown, E.N.; Ronda, J.M.; Kronauer, R.E.; Richardson, G.S.; and Freitag, W.D. 1985. A clinical method to assess the endogenous circadian phase (ECP) of the deep circadian oscillator in man. *Sleep Research* 14:295.

Czeisler, C.A.; Chiasera, A.J.; and Duffy, J.F. 1991. Research on sleep, circadian rhythms, and aging: Applications to manned spaceflight. *Experimental Gerontology* 26:217-232.

Czeisler, C.A.; Johnson, M.P.; Duffy, J.F.; Brown, E.N.; Ronda, J.M.; and Kronauer, R.E. 1990. Exposure to bright light and darkness to treat physiologic maladaptation to night work. *New England Journal of Medicine* 322(18):1253-1259.

Czeisler, C.A.; Moore-Ede, M.C.; and Coleman, R.M. 1982. Rotating shift work schedules that disrupt sleep are improved by applying circadian principles. *Science* 217:460-463.

DeBacker, G.; Kornitzer, M.; Peters, H.; and Dramaix, M. 1984. Relation between work rhythm and coronary risk factors. *European Heart Journal* 5 (supplement 1):307.

Dement, W.C. and Kleitman, N. 1957. The relation of eye move-ments during sleep to dream activity: An objective method of the study of dreaming. *Journal of Experimental Psychology* 53:339-346.

DeVries-Griever, A.H.G. and Meijman, T.F. 1987. The impact of abnormal hours of work on various modes of information pro-cessing: A process model on human costs of performance. *Ergonomics* 30:1287-1299.

Dinges, D.F. 1989. Napping patterns and effects in human adults. In *Sleep and alertness: Chronobiological, behavioral, and medical aspects of napping*, eds. D.F. Dinges and R.J. Broughton, pp. 171-204. New York: Raven Press.

Dinges, D.F. and Broughton, R.J., eds. 1989. *Sleep and alertness: Chronobiological, behavioral, and medical aspects of napping*. New York: Raven Press.

Dyer, J. 1993. Get rid of H. pylori; get rid of ulcer for good? *American Journal of Nursing* 93:47-48.

Eliopoulos, C. 1984. Time management: A reminder. *Journal of Nurs-ing Administration* 4(3):30-32.

Estryn-Behar, M.; Kaminski, M.; Peigne, E.; Bonnet, N.; Vaichere, E.; Gozlan, C.; Azoulay, S.; and Giorgi, M. 1990. Stress at work and mental health status among female hospital workers. *British Journal of Industrial Medicine* 47:20-28.

Folkard, S. 1975. Diurnal variation in logical reasoning. *British Jour-nal of Psychology* 66:1-8.

Folkard, S. and Condon, R. 1987. Night shift paralysis in air traffic control officers. *Ergonomics* 30:1353-1363.

Folkard, S.; Condon, R.; and Herbert, M. 1984. Nightshift paralysis. *Experientia* 40:510-512.

Folkard, S. and Monk, T.H. 1979. Shiftwork and performance. *Human Factors* 21:483-492.

_____. 1985. Circadian performance rhythms. In *Hours of work: Tem-poral factors in work scheduling*, eds. S. Folkard and T.H. Monk, pp. 37-52. New York: John Wiley & Sons.

Folkard, S; Monk, T.H.; Bradbury, R.; and Rosenthall, J. 1977. Time of day effects in school children's immediate and delayed recall of meaningful material. *British Journal of Psychology* 68:45-50.

Folkard, S.; Monk, T.H.; and Lobban, M.C. 1978. Short- and long-term adjustment of circadian rhythms in "permanent" night nurses. *Ergonomics* 21:785-799.

_____. 1979. Towards a predictive test of adjustment to shiftwork. *Ergonomics* 22:79-91.

Foret, J.; Bensimon, G.; Benoit, O.; and Vieux, N. 1981. Quality of sleep as a function of age and shift work. In *Night and shift work: Biological and social aspects*, eds. A. Reinberg, N. Vieux, and P. Andlauer, pp. 149-160. Oxford: Pergamon Press.

Fort, A. and Mills, J.N. 1976. Der Einflub der Tageszeit und des vorherge-henden Schlaf-Wach-Musters auf die Leistungs-Fahig-keit unmittelbar nach dem Aufstehen. In *Biologische Rhythmen und Arbeit*, ed. G. Hilderbrandt. Berlin: Springer-Verlag.

Gadbois, C. 1981. Women on night shift: Interdependence of sleep and off-the-job activities. In *Night and shift work: Biological and social aspects*, eds. A. Reinberg, N. Vieux, and P. Andlauer, pp. 223-227. Oxford: Pergamon Press.

Gold, D.R.; Rogacx, S.; Bock, N.; Tostesm, T.D.; Baum, T.M.; Speizer, F.F.; and Czeisler, C.A. 1992. Rotating shift work, sleep, and accidents related to sleepiness in hospital nurses. *American Journal of Public Health* 82:1011-1014.

Gordon, N.P.; Cleary, P.D.; Parker, C.E.; and Czeisler, C.A. 1986. The prevalence and health impactof shiftwork. *American Journal of Public Health* 76:1225-1228.

Halberg, F. 1969. Chronobiology. *Annual Review of Physiology* 31:675-725.

Hamelin, P. 1987. Lorry drivers' time habits in work and their involvement in traffic accidents. *Ergonomics* 30:1323-1333.

Harma, M.; Ilmarinen, J.; and Knauth, P. 1988. Physical fitness and other individual factors relating to the shiftwork tolerance of women. *Chronobiology International* 5:417-424.

Hauri, P. 1982. *The sleep disorders*. Kalamazoo, Mich.: Upjohn.

Hawkins, L.H. and Armstrong-Esther, C.A. 1978. Circadian rhythms and night shift working in nurses. *Nursing Times* 74(13):49-52.

Hildebrandt, G.; Rohmert, W.; and Rutenfranz, J. 1974. Twelve- and 24-hour rhythms in error frequency of locomotive drivers and the influence of tiredness. *International Journal of Chronobiology* 2:175-180.

Hockey, G.R.J. and Colquhoun, W.P. 1972. Diurnal variation in human performance: A review. In *Aspects of human efficiency: Diurnal rhythm and loss of sleep,* ed. W.P. Colquhoun, pp. 39-107. London: English Universities Press.

Hockey, G.R.J.; Davies, S.; and Gray, M.M. 1972. Forgetting as a function of sleep at different times of day. *Quarterly Journal of Experimental Psychology* 24:389-393.

Horne, J.A. 1988. *Why we sleep: The functions of sleep in humans and other mammals.* Oxford: Oxford University Press.

_____. 1991. Dimensions to sleepiness. In *Sleep, sleepiness and performance,* ed. T.H. Monk, pp. 169-196. Chichester, England: John Wiley & Sons.

Horne, J.A. and Ostberg, O. 1976. A self-assessment questionnaire to determine morningness-eveningness in human circadian rhythms. *International Journal of Chronobiology* 4:97-110.

Hughes, D.G. and Folkard, S. 1976. Adaptation to an 8 h shift in living routine by members of a socially isolated community. *Nature* 264: 432-434.

Jamal, M. and Jamal, S.M. 1982. Work and nonwork experience of employees on fixed and rotating shifts: An empirical assessment. *Journal of Vocational Behavior* 20:282-293.

Jones, D.C.; Bonito, A.J.; Gower, S.C.; and Williams, R.L. 1987. *Analysis of the environment for the recruitment and retention of registered nurses in nursing homes.* Washington, D.C.: U.S. Department of Health and Human Services, Public Health Service, Health Resources and Services Administration.

Kemp, J. 1984. Nursing at night. *Journal of Advanced Nursing* 9:217-223.

Klein, K.E.; Wegmann, H.M.; and Hunt, B.I. 1972. Desynchronization of body temperature and performance circadian rhythms as a result of out-going and home-going transmeridian flights. *Aerospace Medicine* 43(2):119-132.

Kleinsmith, L.J. and Kaplan, S. 1963. Paired-associate learning as a function of arousal and interpolated interval. *Journal of Experimental Psychology* 65:190-193.

Kleitman, N. 1960. The sleep cycle. *American Journal of Nursing* 60:677-679.

_____. 1963. *Sleep and wakefulness,* 2nd ed. Chicago: University of Chicago Press.

Knauth, P.; Emde, E.; Rutenfranz, J.; Kiesswetter, E.; and Smith, P.A. 1981. Re-entrainment of body temperature in field studies of shift work. *International Archives of Occupational and Environmental Health* 49:137-149.

Knutsson, A.; Akerstedt, T.; Jonsson, B.G.; and Orth-Gomer, K. 1986. Increased risk of ischaemic heart disease in shift workers. *Lancet* 12(July):89-92.

Kogi, K. 1985. Introduction to the problems of shift work. In *Hours of work: Temporal factors in work scheduling,* eds. S. Folkard and T.H. Monk, pp. 165-184. Chichester, England: John Wiley & Sons.

Kostreva, M.M. and Genevier, P. 1989. Nurse preferences vs. circadian rhythms in scheduling. *Nursing Management* 20(7):50-62.

Kuchinski, B.B. 1989. The effects of shift work on the menstrual characteristics of nurses. Doctoral dissertation, Johns Hopkins University, Baltimore.

Lavie, P. 1980. The search for cycles in mental performance from Lombard to Kleitman. *Chronobiologia* 7:247-256.

Lewy, A.J.; Sack, R.L.; Miller, L.S.; Hoban, T.M.; Singer, C.M.; Samples, J.R.; and Drauss, G.L. 1986. The use of plasma melatonin levels and light in the assessment and treatment of chronobiologic sleep and mood disorders. *Journal of Neural Transmission* 21(supplement):311-322.

Lewy, A.J.; Wehr, T.A.; Goodwin, F.K.; Newsome, D.A.; and Markey, S.P. 1980. Light suppresses melatonin secretion in humans. *Science* 210:1267-1269.

Mamalle, N.; Lauman, B.; and Lazar, P. 1984. Prematurity and occupational activity during pregnancy. *American Journal of Epidemiology* 119:309-322.

McDonald, A.D.; McDonald, J.C.; Armstrong, B.; Cherry, N.M.; Nolin, A.D.; and Robert, D. 1988. Prematurity and work in pregnancy. *British Journal of Industrial Medicine* 45:56-62.

McLaughlin, B. and Mohr, P. 1988. Approaches to shift work in non-nursing occupations and nursing. In *Secretary's Commission on Nursing final report, vol. 2: Support studies and background information*, XIII, pp. 1-13. Washington, D.C.: U.S. Department of Health and Human Services.

McMurtry, D.E. 1992. *1990 hospital nursing personnel survey: Executive summary*. Chicago: American Hospital Association.

Mellor, E.F. 1986. Shift work and flexitime: How prevalent are they? *Monthly Labor Review* 109:14-21.

Mendelson, W.B. 1987. *Human sleep: Research and clinical care*. New York: Plenum Medical Book Co.

Mills, J.N.; Minors, D.S.; and Waterhouse, J.M. 1978. The effects of sleep upon human circadian rhythms. *Chronobiologia* 5:14-27.

Mitler, M.M.; Carskadon, M.A.; Czeisler, C.A.; Dement, W.C.; Dinges, D.F.; and Graeber, R.C. 1988. Catastrophes, sleep and public policy: Consensus report. *Sleep* 11(1):100-109.

Monk, T.H. 1979. Temporal effects in visual search. In *Search and the human observer*, eds. J.N. Clare and M.A. Sinclair, pp. 30-39. London: Taylor & Francis.

_____. 1986. Advantages and disadvantages of rapidly rotating shift schedules: A circadian viewpoint. *Human Factors* 28:553-557.

_____. 1988. *How to make shift work safe and productive*. Des Plaines, Ill.: American Society of Safety Engineers.

Monk, T.H. and Folkard, S. 1978. Concealed inefficiency of late-night study. *Nature* 273:296-297.

_____. 1992. *Making shift work tolerable*. London: Taylor & Francis.

Monk, T.H.; Fookson, J.E.; Kream, J.; Moline, M.L.; Pollak, C.P.; and Weitzman, M.B. 1985. Circadian factors during sustained performance: Background and methodology. *Behavior Research Methods, Instruments and Computers* 17:19-26.

Moore, R.Y. 1982. The suprachiasmatic nucleus and the organization of a circadian system. *Trends in Neurosciences* 5(11):404-407.

Moore-Ede, M.C. and Richardson, G.S. 1985. Medical implications of shift-work. *Annual Review of Medicine* 36:607-617.

Moore-Ede, M.C.; Sulzman, F.M.; and Fuller, C.A. 1982. *The clocks that time us*. Boston: Harvard University Press.

Moses, E.B. 1990. *The registered nurse population: Findings from the national sample survey of registered nurses, March 1988*. Washington, D.C.: U.S. Department of Health and Human Services, Public Health Service, Health Resources and Services Administration, Division of Nursing.

Mott, P.E.; Mann, F.C.; McLoughlin, Q.; and Warwick, D.P. 1965. *Shift work: The social, psychological, and physical consequences.* Ann Arbor, Mich.: University of Michigan Press.

Neylan, T.C. and Reynolds, C.F. 1991. Pathological sleepiness. In *Sleep, sleepiness and performance,* ed. T.H. Monk, pp. 199-222. Chichester, England: John Wiley & Sons.

Panel investigates effects of shift rotation. May 1983. *The American Nurse,* p. 3.

Patkai, P. 1971. Interindividual differences in diurnal variations in alertness, performance, and adrenaline excretion. *Acta Physiologica Scandinavica* 81:35-46.

Presser, H.B. 1987. Work shifts of full-time dual earner couples: Patterns and contrasts by sex of spouse. *Demography* 24:99-112.

Prokop, O. and Prokop, L. 1955. Ermunudung und Einschlafen am Steuer. *Zentralblatt fur Verkehrs-Medizin, Verkehrs-Psychologie und angrenzende Gebiete* 1:19-30.

Rechtschaffen, A. and Kales, A.A. 1968. *A manual of standardized terminology, techniques, and scoring system for sleep stages of human subjects.* Bethesda, Md.: National Institute of Neurological Diseases and Blindness.

Reinberg, A.; Vieux, N.; and Andlauer, P. 1981. *Night and shift: Biological and social aspects.* Oxford: Pergamon Press.

Rusak, B. 1977. The role of the suprachiasmatic nuclei in the generation of circadian rhythms in the golden hamster, Mesocricetus auratus. *Journal of Comparative Physiology* 118:145-146.

Rutenfranz, J. 1982. Occupational health measures for night- and shiftworkers. *Journal of Human Ergology* 11 (supplement):67-86.

Rutenfranz, J.; Colquhoun, W.P.; Knauth, P.; and Ghata, J.N. 1977. Biomedical and psychosocial aspects of shift-work. *Scandinavian Journal of Work, Environment, and Health* 3:165-182.

Rutenfranz, J.; Haider, M.; and Koller, M. 1985. Occupational health measures for nightworkers and shiftworkers. In *Hours of work: Temporal factors in work scheduling,* eds. S. Folkard and T.H. Monk, pp. 199-210. New York: John Wiley & Sons.

Scherrer, J. 1981. Man's work and circadian rhythm through the ages. In *Night and shift work: Biological and social aspects,* eds. A. Reinberg, N. Vieux, and P. Andlauer, pp. 1-10. Oxford: Pergamon Press.

Schwirian, P. 1978. Evaluating the performance of nurses: A multidimensional approach. *Nursing Research* 27:347-351.

Scott, A.J. and LaDou, J. 1990. Shiftwork: Effects on sleep and health with recommendations for medical surveillance and screening. *Occupational Medicine* 5:273-299.

Severino, S.K. and Moline, M.L. 1989. *Premenstrual syndrome: A clinician's guide.* New York: Guilford Press.

Singer, G. 1989. Women and shiftwork. In *Managing shiftwork,* ed. M. Wallace, pp. 25-48. Bundoora, Australia: Brain-Behavior Research Institute.

Skipper, J.K.; Jung, F.D.; and Coffey, L.C. 1990. Nurses and shiftwork: Effects on physical health and mental depression. *Journal of Advanced Nursing* 15:835-842.

Smolensky, M.H. and Reinberg, A. 1990. Clinical chronobiology: Relevance and applications to the practice of occupational medicine. *Occupational Medicine* 5:239-272.

Staines, G.L. and Pleck, J.H. 1984. Nonstandard work schedules and family life. *Journal of Applied Psychology* 69:515-523.

Tasto, D.L. and Colligan, M.J. 1978. *Health consequences of shift work.* Menlo Park, Calif.: Stanford Research Institute.

Teleky, L. 1943. Problems of night work: Influences on health and efficiency. *Industrial Medicine* 12:758-779.

Tepas, D.I. and Carvalhais, A.B. 1990. Sleep patterns of shift workers. *Occupational Medicine* 5:199-208.

Tepas, D.I.; Walsh, J.K.; and Armstrong, D.R. 1981. Comprehensive study of the sleep of shiftworkers. In *The twenty-four hour workday: Proceedings of a symposium on variations in work-sleep schedules,* eds. L.C. Johnson, D.I. Tepas, W.P. Colquhoun, and M.J. Colligan, pp. 419-433. Cincinnati: U.S. Department of Health and Human Services, National Institute of Occupational Safety and Health.

U.S. Congress, Office of Technology Assessment. 1991. *Biological rhythms: Implications for the worker.* Washington, D.C.: U.S. Government Printing Office.

Uehata, T. and Sasakawa, N. 1982. The fatigue and maternity disturbances of night workwomen. *Journal of Human Ergology* 11(supplement):465-474.

Verhaegen, P.; Cober, P.; De Smedt, M.; Dirkx, J.; Kerstens, J.; Ryvers, D.; and Van Daele, P. 1987. The adaptation of night nurses to different work schedules. *Ergonomics* 30:1301-1309.

Walker, J.M. 1985. Social problems of shift work. In *Hours of work: Temporal factors in work scheduling,* eds. S. Folkard and T.H. Monk, pp. 211-225. New York: John Wiley & Sons.

Walsh, J.K.; Muehlbach, M.J.; and Schweitzer, P.K. 1984. Acute administration of triazolam for the daytime sleep of rotating shift workers. *Sleep* 7:223-229.

Wehr, T.A. and Goodwin, F.K. 1983. *Circadian rhythms in psychiatry.* Pacific Grove, Calif.: Boxwood.

Weitzman, E.D.; Czeisler, C.A.; and Moore-Ede, M.C. 1979. Sleep-wake, neuroendocrine, and body temperature circadian rhythms under entrained and non-entrained (free-running) conditions in man. In *Biological rhythms and their central mechanisms,* eds. M. Suda, O. Hayaishi, and H. Nakagawa, pp. 199-227. Amsterdam: Elsevier.

Wever, R.A. 1975. The circadian multi-oscillator system of man. *International Journal of Chronobiology* 3:19-55.

———. 1979. *The circadian system of man: Results of experiments under temporal isolation.* New York: Springer-Verlag.

Wilkinson, R. and Allison, S. 1989. Alertness of night nurses: Two shift-systems compared. *Ergonomics* 32:281-292.

Wojtczak-Jaroszowa, J. and Pawlowska-Skyba, K. 1967. Night and shift work: Circadian variations in work. *Medycyna Pracy* 18:1.